To All Those: "Who Run Where the Brave Dare Not Go." ~ From: "The Impossible Dream, ('Man of La Mancha' Musical)

Table of Contents

Extended and Cryptic Pregnancy Midwife

The First Work of its Kind, that Charts, Describes and Observes the Extended and Cryptic Pregnancy Phenomenon

By, Anshin B. Kelly, TM, ECPM, WMP
Traditional Midwife, Extended and Cryptic Pregnancy Midwife, Wilderness Medicine Practitioner

Traditional Midwifery is Protected Under the First Amendment

Why Traditional Midwifery is Vulnerable to Chronic Persecution, even though it has been Long Sanctioned Under Basic American Freedoms

The one thing that differentiates Traditional Midwifery from any other kind of Modern Midwifery that are regulated through various Federal as well as State Laws and legal obligations, is this: **Traditional Midwifery is inherently grounded in Spiritual/Religious Cultural Identity and Tradition.**

The First Amendment of the United States Constitution:

AMENDMENT I

"Congress shall make no law respecting an establishment of religion,

or prohibiting the free exercise thereof; or abridging the freedom of speech, or of the press; or the right of the people peaceably to assemble, and to petition the Government for a redress of grievances."

Traditional Midwives around the world are predominantly trained through mentorship with senior midwives and self-teaching. They choose to continue this way of life, even after centuries of severe persecution, for one major reason only:

Traditional Midwifery is rooted in the foundational belief, that childbirth, motherhood, and family, are inherently Spiritual, not medical in nature. Traditional Midwifery is, and has been for thousands of years, inextricably tied to Spiritual/Religious structures and beliefs.

Traditional Midwives do not consider pregnancy and childbirth to be "medical conditions." Pregnancy and childbirth are a fundamental part of human life, and Nature Itself has an inherent Wisdom, Authority, and yes, _Godliness_ in this matter.

As Traditional Midwives, and the mothers choosing our care, we have the inherent Constitutional Freedom to practice, and receive Traditional Midwifery Care.

Of course, this clashes severely, as always to Federal Tax Laws. A Traditional Midwife deserves to receive a living wage for her work, and I am not suggesting that she is automatically now "Tax Exempt," like a Church. However, the Federal Government and the "Powers that Be," tend to extort the ignorance of the easily intimidated everyday person, and create an intimidating illusion that Federal Law is a solid, stone statue that never changes. That never has to readdress important matters (such as the Ancient Practice of Traditional Midwifery). When, contrary to systemic everyday belief, the Federal Government is constantly having to readdress laws, and various issues that crop up on every layer of Government, and Law; and most importantly, rethink, and reassess these issues' relationship to the bedrock of our American Freedoms and Laws: The US Constitution.

The severe persecution of Traditional Midwives continues unbroken in the West, since at least the 15th Century. I have seen Traditional Midwives, who became the Pillars of their respective communities, cut-down by legal attacks and severe thrashings, that are too often supported by middle/upper-class hysteria; due to predominantly Medical, White, Western Male (and now Female), propaganda, that has also gone on, unbroken since at least the eighteenth century; against the long-standing, and Sacred Practice of Traditional Midwifery.

This is my "redress of grievances," exercised through Constitutional Free Speech. The Bill of Rights also protects citizens from undue, excessive punishment and cruelty. Totally legitimate, and Expert Traditional Midwives in America have gone and chained themselves to red tape, simply because they fear the hysteria that threw their fellow Traditional Midwives headlong into the social flames of a pyre, built by her persecutors, and supported predominantly, by social, widespread hysteria. This kind of pattern, inflicted over and over again, is absolutely, excessive and cruel, and therefore Unconstitutional; and therefore, as I am a Traditional Midwife, inherently governed by Higher Law, I proclaim it also, an Attack on the Human Spirit, and therefore immoral.

Traditional Midwives are therefore the only Professional Women, and indeed *people in a society* who can powerfully and effectively protect the Basic Human and Civil Rights of All People! We protect Human Life (All People) from its Inception and Women, through both Moral and Civil Law. It is therefore only rational, and self-evident that The First Amendment is our Core Legal Platform and Pivot Point;

as The First Amendment unapologetically proclaims the

Legal Freedoms of both Civil and Moral Matters.

I think we are beginning to see why the persecution of Traditional Midwifery has been so long-standing: The Traditional Midwife, since Ancient Times, is extremely Spiritually powerful, and not technically ever under ANY absolute jurisdiction or control.

A person such as this, has never been easily tolerated by "The Powers that Be," both secular and religious. Indeed, A Person such as this, is often easily, and severely subject to persecution, from both secular and religious factions.

Anshin B. Kelly, Traditional Midwife, and
Wilderness Medicine Practitioner.

A Note to Medical Professionals:

I have taken great care in this write up to try and strike a profound balance between stating from my lived experience, the collective experiences of hundreds of women I have worked with, what I have seen as the grave failures of the medical field in regards to women's health both historically and currently; As well as my acknowledgement of the great potential, dignity and legacy and accomplishments of the Western Scientific realm.

From my perspective; the truth must be stated. No matter the potential, and in many ways, inescapable reality that feelings will be hurt and long-held beliefs challenged. Women and babies have lost their lives, and at the very least, have been deeply traumatized and broken through the consistent denial of the cryptic pregnancy and extended gestation phenomenon. I've seen and experienced this reality with my own eyes, ears, heart and all my senses for the last almost a decade. Angering some medical professionals is, in my opinion, a very small price to pay for the lives of babies and mothers lost.

My hope is that you'll see my great desire to gradually come to work symbiotically with the medical field as a Traditional Healer and Midwife. Together, I profoundly believe that we can help many more women find better balance, health and peace in their lives. To me, personal feelings do not matter when so much is at stake.

Facing the Fire: Saint Joan of Arc, Mother of CP/EG and the Modern Woman

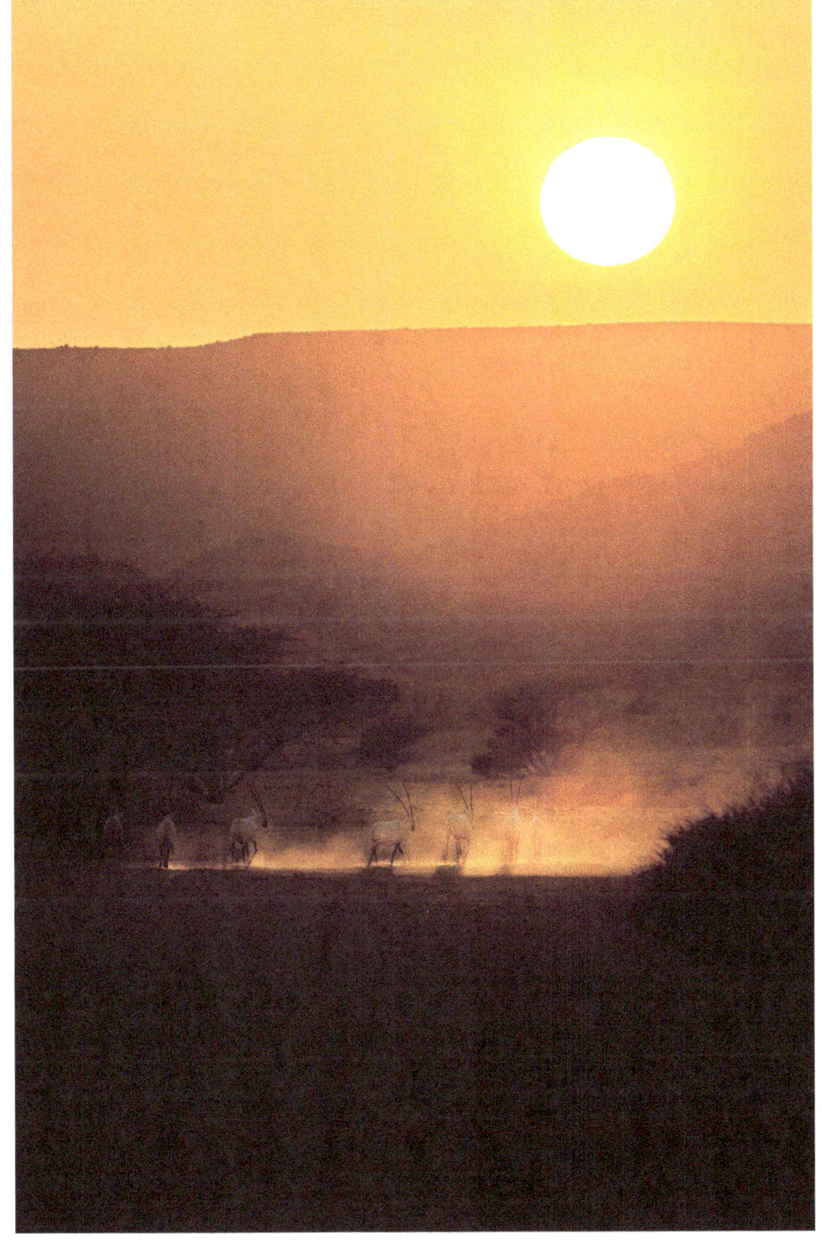

"Now the flames they followed Joan of Arc
As she came riding through the dark
No moon to keep her armor bright
No man to get her through this very smoky night

She said, 'I'm tired of the war
I want the kind of work I had before
A wedding dress or something white
To wear upon my swollen appetite...'

...And deep into his fiery heart
he took the dust of Joan of Arc,
and high above the wedding guests
he hung the ashes of her wedding dress...

...I saw the glory in her eye.
Myself I long for love and light,
but must it come so cruel, and oh so bright?"

~ Leonard Cohen, "Joan of Arc"

The Passing of Obasan's Bones

This memory is so sacred, that I asked Obasan's Spirit, (my paternal grandmother) if I could tell it. Not only did she give her blessing, but I feel she is the one who gave me the idea in the first place.

When I was a very small child, between three and five years old, our family traveled to Japan to attend the burial rituals and ceremonies of my Obasan. I don't remember almost anything about that trip, except for a few radiant scraps here and there, that I get mixed up I think perhaps with my Ojisan's burial.

What I remember are The Bones. In Japanese culture, there is an ancient ritual in which the family gathers around the cremated remains of the recently deceased ancestor. There is a huge, sacred urn that is used for the bones and ashes, and is then taken home and placed on the altar at the house. Using special chopsticks, each family member, one at a time, will select a bone to be passed all around the entire family circle, to finally end at the urn, and be placed in it.

I was watching everything with absolute wonderment. Right near me, to my right, I saw the skull buried slightly in the ashes. I knew, when it came my turn I was going to choose it for my bone to pass around the circle. When it came my turn, I took both my chopsticks and I stuck them both inside the skull, and began to lift it.

I remember, very clearly, no one discouraged me from doing this; a tiny girl lifting her ancestor's skull with chopsticks. I remember the skull slipped slightly and in an instant, eight or nine pairs of chopsticks appeared around the skull to help. The relatives now attached to the skull with me, helped to slowly guide it ever so respectfully, and gently, into the urn.

~ Anshin B Kelly

Joan of Arc is a respected, female Saint in the Catholic Tradition. She is also a historical figure, and French heroine who lived during the fifteenth century. Her history recalls her calling from God as a young teenager to prepare herself in body and soul to one day lead a French army to victory against the British. This she did, in her late teens, a lowly commoner and peasant girl, who convinced the dethroned French ruler at the time to let her do it.

Her victories led to France's liberation from their colonizers. Eventually she was captured by the British, tried with witchcraft, and murdered through stake burning. However, as soon as a mere handful of decades later after her murder, the books concerning her trial and sentencing were reopened, deeply questioned and eventually given proper, albeit terribly belated exoneration.

Joan of Arc has also been a lifelong guardian and spiritual mother in my life; and even having to hear and process the horrific endings of her physical life, spiritually, this only served to help me face the "fires" of my own unspeakable torments starting from when I was very young.

I truly feel that Mama Joan, like so many people who suffered unspeakably, and were able to pass through those trials to come out the other side and in a deeply spiritual sense, "reclaim the soul fires" that were taken and used by predator forces to hurt them; because she triumphed, would like women (and men), to meditate on her life, trials, torments and victories, in a symbolic and spiritual sense. It was through the torments of my life, and also the processing of Mama Joan's life, that I came to the unshakable knowing and realization, that the physical aspects of torment should not be dwelt upon. Remembering them has its place, but it should be minimal. Instead, we need to focus on what spiritually powerful people have to teach us through initiation in an emotional, psychological, and spiritual sense. *This doesn't make it easier mind you, but it helps us to put focus and attention on solutions, rather than terror, and unresolved pain.*

The First Wedding Dress

"After ten years of relationship with my husband and 8 years of marriage and four children later, I wanted to pass this on to you;

It's really very true that Love, True Love, has rhythmical periods of peace, radiant and deep, deep comfort and contentment; as well as storms, trials and sometimes vast valleys and peaks to climb/ scramble/sometimes tumble down, landing no less on one's face at times!

Something that goes deeply hand in hand with the above is something that isn't as spoken of, and therefore perhaps able to avoid getting lost in a cliche, it's deep meaning overlooked. And it is this;

True Love shows up in times we are tested, in the guise of something really, not so pretty, maybe even revolting at first appearances, and maybe even considered 'mean.' True Love will ask for her wounds to be kissed and licked, soothed and bandaged. She'll ask you to carry her, raw and infected wounds and all, over a raging river. If you're like most of us, well then there's going to be times you run screaming from the ugliness, forgetting completely that True Love, not just emotions, not just love tied up in a hashtag...True Love, the love that overcomes anything, that is there, with her inconveniences, her unconventional 'mean' 'harsh' solutions, her silent ways, her 'dark' ways, and on the other hand, her deep, deep endless compassion, forgiveness and wisdom, IS TEACHER. AND THEREFORE, TEACHING YOU. Teaching you what? How to listen. How.To.Listen. To what? To no less than the SOUL. The Soul knows; what to keep and what to let go, what to let live and what to let die, even sever, if need be. And last but not least, HOW TO FACE THE DARKNESS, WITH YOUR LIGHT.

Listen deep, and learn to recognize True Love in her many guises and she'll deepen you, your lives and your marriage beyond your VERY WILDEST dreams.

All my Love, Anshin"

It's time to gather around The Bones.

I wrote the above quote in an email to some young women at the time, who seemed to be in the flurries of euphoric wedding preparations. They never answered back, and now that it think about it, of course it could have been chalked up to the fact that they were in a flurry of wedding preparations, and, not to mention the sweet, sweet beginnings of new, and budding love; however, their wedding was delayed a full year, and they answered pretty much every other email I sent. I don't wish to run speculation beyond appropriate boundaries, however, deep inside my heart, as an experienced woman, wife, mother and midwife, I know why they never responded.

The first wedding dress is, in this life on earth -perhaps if it were a different earth it would not be- both new love, and the capture and imprisonment of that love. The Sacred Feminine is "The Gateway" for all humankind; her first marriage initiation, whether spiritual or physical and both, symbolized in the wedding dress, will be both love and a torment of that love.

As also a pretty active and ever-growing historian and theologian, I have never seen anyone able to avoid this pattern; even or especially in the holiest and best of life circumstances and blessings. However, the naive initiate, always, even desperately, hopes that this ain't so.

I feel deeply that this is why divorce rates are so high in modernized cultures at large, and "marriages" and/ or relationships of more comfort, fear of being alone, and convenience are formed rampantly in this culture at large.

The modern person is conditioned to run from the fire, and at times comes back only after someone or something else has taken the fall- for their escape from accountability, and soul initiation- and they are signaled by the dark forces or "puppeteers" of modernism, to desecrate the annihilation site, instead of facing it.

Most CP/EG mothers I have met and intimately worked with, have spent years running from the fire. Mama Joan faced the fires when she accepted her mission from Spirit, at a very tender young age. Her physical death was only one of the times she did, and for her I feel deeply, wasn't even the most important/prominent fire-facing. Her physical death was a crime against the Soul, not an initiation unto itself. However, even in the most desperate of circumstances, Spirit has the transcendent power of initiation and transformation. Most CP/EG mothers will also have times in which they did face the Soul-Fire in their lives, but later bought into the relative distractions and comforts of the modernistic mind, and ego. The reasons why I know this are pretty numerous, however, I would say that one of the reasons I know is most likely the most primary, and that is: They are content to wear their initial Soul Initiation as a badge, instead of understanding it as the narrow entryway, or pass, through which we become able to pass through Soul-Fires not once, twice or three times…but as a way of life, until we are one with it; as in oneness of Body and Soul.

The "first wedding dress" symbolizes not only our purity, but also our immaturity. It symbolizes our joyful, natural and childlike zest for life, and it also symbolizes our unrealistic, and inexperienced expectations. One thing is for absolute certainty; the first wedding dress serves her purpose.

She holds every first, every fiber of pure hope, happiness, and unconditional love that flows freely from children. She bears also the marks of the firsts that hurt us, shocked us, left us, betrayed us. She is there to carry us over many significant thresholds that help to "marry" us and bind to, or ground us into our earthly lives. She is the Spiritual Protector, and aspect of the Sacred Feminine, who is with us, and embraces us through natural, as well as harsher, human instigated Initiations.

But there comes a time when the Soul-Fire must consume Her, so that the initiate wearing the first wedding dress can pass through to the next stage of Soul growth and passage to greater awareness and deeper knowing.

There comes a time a woman and/or a CP/EG mother, begins to feel hunger, or "a swollen appetite," because certain experiences have driven her to Soul-Calling in a deeper form, and she finds herself winning many battles for herself, and perhaps those around her, but nonetheless, the more she fights forward to victory, the more unusable and inadequate the first wedding dress, who has served her so righteously this far, becomes; for those battles and victories are serving a greater purpose far beyond the immediate mission and journey.

It's time to face the Soul-Fire. To let it burn all that came before; all the perceived "good" and the "bad," all the triumphs, and the "badges," and all the perceived failures, it's time to allow Reclamation to happen.

The Soul's Kiln of Transformation

Most modern women in my experience not only run from the slightest sensation of heat, but they perceive the heat immediately as a threat to their most current, "inmost" identity, or something even more terrifying than that, *failure*. Failure for the modern woman is often, in a lot of ways, worse than physical death. I've seen too many throughout my life end their lives, rather than face their difficult circumstances, and/or mistakes.

In many other cases, failure is so unbearable to the modern woman, she'd rather succumb to a competitive, ruthless mentality, especially towards other women, rather than face her

Soul's Kiln of Transformation.

In my experience, the modern woman has more filthy, blood, and other stained, torn "first" wedding gowns in her phycological closet, than her great grandmother, and grandmother's going back generations ever did; and yet, she scorns the women who came before her for their perceived "subservience" to their husbands or other male superiors and counterparts, and resents history bitterly for the times women were held down, tried, and even murdered unjustly, and with impunity.

This is all completely understandable. However, the cold, bitterness that rules, jeers, and blocks entry to feminine annihilation sites psychologically, and many times physically, in the modern age, for decades, has been primarily fueled by females.

A woman can not truly move forward and become initiated without knowing how to face the fire. Throughout most of ancient history, women had a continuous legacy in place, passed from grandmother to mother to daughter, on The Way of Feminine Soul-Fire Initiation. Indeed, the mythos, teachings, traditional rites and folklore of ancient traditions since time out of mind, all around the world, have taught the core existence, and reality of the Soul's Kiln of Transformation; and women primarily, were the keepers and bequestors of this ancient wisdom and rites of passage.

Maybe we have a whole walk-in closet, or hell, several, or double hell, maybe whole storage units filled with filthy, hidden and therefore neglected first wedding dresses. Maybe we just have one, but either way, if it was hung up somewhere instead of submitted to Soul-Fire, then our work is to deeply examine why we won't, and/or can't relinquish the past, and all it's everything in every way, to the Will of the Soul, and instead cling to it; and bite, mock, assault, or manipulate anyone who wants, consciously or unconsciously, to help us see these unhealthy, and even extremely toxic patterns in our lives.

A kiln has been used for thousands of years as a way of transforming, solidifying, and/or annihilating something in a permanent way.

One time I made a sea- turtle-jewelry-dish out of clay. It was made up of a bottom dish, and a top cover, and the bottom was the chest-plate-shell, fins, head and tail of the turtle, and the cover was the top, domed shell. It was a demanding project, but I did it with not much trouble at all, and with a lot of joy, and pride. It was to be a gift to a young woman and fellow counselor at a summer camp.

I added pigments to my turtle before putting it into the kiln, to harden, and to cure the colors onto the surface of the clay.

When my turtle dish emerged from the kiln, the art teacher and I were absolutely astounded at what we saw: Her fins and tail had become wavy in the extreme heat of the kiln, and it truly looked as if she were swimming! It was absolutely marvelous, and for me, a deeply spiritual experience.

It can be an extremely painful experience to submit that first wedding dress to the Soul-Fire. But that can not be a reason to not do it. Clinging to that first wedding dress only leads to even worse pain, wounding, and sorrow for ourselves, our spouses, our children, our friends, and our communities.

CP/EG mothers who have the hardest time accepting their pregnancies, and the deeply unique, and often immensely challenging natures of their pregnancies, are mostly women in my experience who have more than one first wedding dress hung up somewhere.

One young CP/EG mother I knew years ago, was a mess when it came to the challenging reality of her body and baby, and therefore the impact it was all having on her marriage, and her life in general.

When I look back now, she was desperately clinging to some

fragment of her innocence that had been annihilated at one time in her younger years, through an abortion. When she got married to the man she loved, I can see now she saw it at least subconsciously, as a way to attain another "first" wedding dress, a "cleaner" one, without totally having to face the Soul-Fire regarding the other first wedding dress, and the bloodstains of heartbreak, shame, guilt and disappointment she felt in herself, upon it. At the time I had very little experience in these matters, especially in regards to the modern woman and CP/EG, but I'd submitted many a wedding, and post-wedding/working dress, to Soul-Fire, in my difficult yet, deeply initiated life, from a very young age. I remember in many ways fully submitting again, the current "Soul-Dress" I was wearing, in order to be fully initiated as ECPM (Extended and Cryptic Pregnancy Midwife), which from that time, would take about seven years to complete.

The Mama Sea Turtle, or "Tortuga Mami" I sometimes call her, is a pivotal symbol of the Sacred Feminine. She is Hell, and she is High Water. She is fire and she is water. I find it immeasurably fascinating how in Norse Mythology "Hel" is the name of a pretty deeply misunderstood, in modern times, Goddess figure, and ruler of the land of the dead, in tribal European traditions. It is through my life experiences with "Hel" or what I've come to understand as the"Death in Life" force, and Sacred Feminine, that I came to deeply understand the Soul's Kiln of Transformation.

Woman is The Gateway of Death in Life. Her womb is every Soul's Way of Transformation and Initiation, because every Soul came through a woman.

Passing of the Bones

Modernistic thinking germinated from Euro-Christian radicalized beliefs about the Sacred Feminine, which is the Root Mother of the overall ancient world. Radicalized Euro-Christian beliefs about the Sacred Feminine, and therefore women at large, were instigated to seize control away from the Centers of, since time-out-of-mind, clans and communities in the ancient world, who were, and are still, in many parts of the world, Wise Women Midwives and Healers.

The Wise Woman Midwife and Healer, was where the "rivers" of Death in Life flowed from, and into, in a clan, tribe or community. They were, and are, the Gatekeepers between the worlds of Spirit and Body, namely, the Death in Life Force.

CP/EG women are often women who have dealt with extremely debilitating health issues in their lives, before their CP/EG began. They are often women who have spent their lives enduring varying levels of abuse, and/or have managed to earn some level of social notoriety and/or respect. They are often financially stable, but came up from nothing, and their CP/EG is throwing the most maddening, and crazy "wrench in their gears" of success and social acceptance. *They want their old lives back, and NOW!!! "Dr. Ani, please," they plead with me, in hundreds of varying ways, "give me a pill that will make it all go away..."*

Even in my most bewildered, and doubtful times, I've answered them since the beginning, *"Sorry dear, I don't deal in blue pills, never have."*

"She said, 'I'm tired of the war
I want the kind of work I had before
A wedding dress or something white
To wear upon my swollen appetite…' "

Most, in also hundreds of varying ways, will scream, stomp their little feet, and never call me again.

This "swollen appetite" in modern women, and loss of maternal guidance for and in men, is nothing new, but I do feel that in the modern age, the seduction to succumb to destructive thinking is at an all time high.

In my work with women from all over North America and the globe, it is rare to meet a woman who is willing to first of all, face the Soul-Fire, secondly, gather around the annihilation site, then thirdly, be willing to pass the bones.

The meaning of passing bones is *recognition*. The blood is made in the bone marrow, and primarily processed, cleansed, broken down, protected and renewed through the liver. In other words, in our passing of the bones symbology, and psychological and spiritual healing processes, new creation occurs through facing the Soul-Fire, likened to new blood cells formed in the bone marrow, and passing the bones is likened to the blood being made healthy, and pure through being passed through the wondrous filtration system that is the liver.

The liver is what I've come to understand through my midwifery and healing work, as *The Gatekeeper.* He protects the blood-origin/ Soul-Fire processes in the bone marrow, that I have come to understand as *The Mother.*

Many times when we are led through the Soul-Fires, it is through immense, and intense circumstances, that take all of our energy and focus. Our powers of discernment are being melted down, shaped and formed in that time, but it is not until we see it through to the end, and we gather around the bones that we begin to use those newfound, and rebirthed tools to move on, and move forward.

It is in my experience that even if a modern woman and/or CP/EG mother sees it through the Soul-Fires, it isn't until the next stage, where she must gather around the annihilation site, she faces her deepest challenges, fears and monsters.

Being able to pass the bones around the circle of Eternity-Life/Death/Rebirth- and have each one gently and courageously, with unwavering vigilance, placed back into the Urn of Self-Recognition, of Soul-Rest, is at the essence of what reclamation is.

"First they ignore you,
Then they laugh at you,
Then they fight you,
Then you win."

~ Mahatma Gandhi

The demons that abused the fire to burn you, are now white with rage and panic, because they can not see what the Creator sees; and that this that the Soul is the Fire. So it is ultimately through the annihilation, even parts of it that are totally unjust and abusive, that the Soul totally reclaims power. The demons have to now fight you, and guard the annihilation site, in order to try and prevent you from seeing clearly, the cosmic power of Death in Life, that is made clear through what is left; and those are the bones.

In the soulful, central words of Mahatma Gandhi, "Then they fight you, then, you win," we see that when it is most intense, when things seem the most gutted, the most stripped, the most lost, it is because we are at the threshold of victory; so this tells us one very important thing we must follow through on in order to not lose everything we've suffered for, and that is: *We must not give up.*

The demons, complexes and shadows of doubt, will pull out all the stops to prevent you from making headway to the inner, sacred circle of the annihilation site. They often, as I've seen with many,

many modern and/or CP/EG women, who are at this stage in their soulful initiation, attack the women through family, and/or people close to the women. Many women have succumbed during this stage, and become part of the mob within their own psyches, families or communities, that snarl, and stand in the way of the last stages before a soulful initiation is complete.

The most important thing to remember in this stage is, that we have learned much through the Soul's Kiln of Transformation, we have mightier tools now than we've ever dreamed of before now. The Creator doesn't have us face the annihilation site without first passing through the Soul-Fire, we must remember that we have what it takes now.

We are not alone. We are guarded from being overcome by dark forces. Because we faced the Soul-Fires and emerged triumphant, we now also have foundational tools of discernment; we can make our way through the cold, dark, white rage and panic without being touched, because we now hold the Eternal Flame, and nothing, and no one can take it from us as long as we put our total trust in it.

"I AM the Dark, that Imbues the Light"

The above are words given to me by The Great Mother, or whom I have come to call the Root Mother; The Sacred Feminine and Root Creator.

Mama Joan, through her life and legacy, became one with the Mother Force, as the Dark, the Light, the Water, the Fire, and Death in Life. Without proper understanding of the Sacred Feminine- the Dark Holy Womb from which all life is conceived, born, and reclaimed- the Westernized, modern world will continue to see more delay in awakening to the truth, and therefore more anguish for women, children, men, and every age group.

The Dark that Imbues the Light, is the tomb that transfigures into the womb. Only within the Holy Feminine, and essentially in women, can and does this happen. Men are reborn through the Essential Feminine, if not through true, womanly connection, then through a deep, mystical relationship to the Divine Feminine on a singular, personal level.

The modern woman and/or CP/EG woman, stand at the threshold between the annihilation site, and outer/inner influences. I feel collectively, on many major levels, modern, feminine culture is in the process of passing through the Soul-Fires. Of course many, many are refusing to face the fires to begin with, however, I feel that there is a core group of a courageous few, who have not wavered fundamentally, and are dedicated to seeing our collective feminine initiation through.

Reclamation is the main feminine work. The womb through women, is both the annihilation and reclamation site of all human beings. In the modern age the womb has been sold up-river to the highest bidder. Instead of being central, it is, in overall culture, deeply commoditized, abused, and therefore subject to deep, fundamental neglect.

However things stand now in our lives, it does not, and can not change the fact *that the time is now.* The time is now to rise up against our inner and outer dark forces. If we haven't already in this cycle period of life, whatever or whenever that is, we must begin by facing the Soul-Fire. It's time to remember who we are on the most essential level of our beings, and to realize that we have what it takes for the task of reclamation.

We must face the cold, attacking mob around the annihilation site, and remember that it is at this stage of things that we are actually very near to the completion of our current, and perhaps very first, and therefore hardest initiation.

The modern person has lost the Way of Initiation. We have become sold to distractions and self-gratifications of every kind, and still more variations on every kind of distraction variation.

CP/EG mothers are called to a very deep work, and that work is the Way of Initiation. Rebirth occurs through the womb, and the reclaiming of the annihilated recognition, and connection of Soul to Body, which is immeasurable reverence for all life,

And an unshakable trust in Death in Life.

Introduction

I am alleging that major and medically-sourced websites such as WebMD, American Pregnancy, and Healthline, and the like are farming and stealing my intellectual property and work regarding the Cryptic Pregnancy and Extended Gestation Experience. It is my most ardent intention to illustrate, that I am the only midwife in all of North America, and probably the Western world, who has the experience, and up to a decade of training, through this experience, on the subject, and therefore the ability to articulate extremely specific, and pivotal observations on the subject.

I am the only midwife that I know of in the published and online world at large who has made connections between things such as nutrition, birth control, uterine trauma (both medical and otherwise), and neglect, and CP/EG. I know that I am the source and sole authorship of the term "CP/EG," (Cryptic Pregnancy and Extended Gestation) and well as "ECPM," (Extended and Cryptic Pregnancy Midwife).

These major medicalized sources and sites routinely do not cite me as their source, and instead, artfully and strategically hide my observational data and written experience in the casual tone of, "this is just common sense." My answer to this manipulative tone is this: If it is just "common sense" extrapolated from thousands of women's experiences with CP/EG, then why, isn't there medically instituted and endorsed prenatal care for these women and their babies?

I own the only childbearing practice in North America that I know of who openly, and publicly and officially includes CP/EG babies and mothers.

My journey with CP/EG began with my second daughter and child, almost a decade ago. I have been in the trenches all these years with hundreds of women from all over the world, who routinely are experiencing at times extreme neglect, ostracism and abuse from trusted medical professionals, their communities and their families.

It's time that credit be given where credit is due, and it goes far beyond me; this has always been about the sanctity of women, babies and life itself. However, citing me as one's source, would be a good place to start.

Other Countries Have Been Way Ahead of the West, for Centuries

Cryptic Pregnancy and Extended Gestation is a relatively well known and accepted phenomenon in places like Africa, India, and other various parts of Asia; specifically in places where the impact of medicalization is less so, and their Traditional Midwifery and Medicine Practices are still intact. There are Traditional Midwives who assist these women and their babies with their pregnancies and births every day. I myself did a full pelvic exam/palpation, and diagnosis of a pregnancy of a Native African woman who was clearly pregnant with around a five pound baby, and who's doctors and husband all denied existence. After her appointment with me, with renewed courage and motherly sense, she went on to travel back to her home country in Africa and get proper care from a Traditional Midwife there, and give birth to a healthy baby. These African Traditional Midwives have shared through their ancestral knowledge, legacy, and experience that their Midwife predecessors have been caring for women with extended gestations since the twelfth century. I did not say "cryptic pregnancy" because "cryptic" pregnancy is a phenomenon that has to a very large extent emerged after the discovery of pregnancy testing through lab work and ultrasound technology.

From a Traditional Healing and Midwife perspective, women and children are first and foremost sacred, not "patients." The womanly intuition has for hundreds of thousands of years been the bedrock on and from which the traditional "sciences" and eventually, in comparison, a fairly "modern" legacy of the Western Sciences have been birthed, cultivated and built. Anthropologists and historians have long concluded that the first and most revered Healers and Midwives were women, and still are, in many areas of the world.

My compilation of in-depth experience, research and discovery is a calling not only in the present, but from somewhere in the ancient and much forgotten past of human healing and birthing knowledge. It is a call to action; both for inward examination of our long-held beliefs and post-modernism, as well as for outward networking, support and powerful change.

"In my experience, it's not that anything and everything is possible, but we are absolutely, without a doubt, sorely ignorant and/or misinformed as a modern, medical society about what *is* actually possible." Anshin Kelly

PART ONE

What is a Cryptic Pregnancy and Extended Gestation? (CP/EG)

A CP/EG is characterized by the fact that the pregnancy can not be (for what I've come to call a "perfect storm"of reasons) medically diagnosed. Some of the main medical reasons for this are the following:

Negative lab test; too low production of HCG, also known as "the pregnancy hormone" for a lab to consider a "viable pregnancy."

Negative sonogram; An unclear picture or inability to spot a baby in a sonogram.

Defensive medicine; In this case, defensive medicine is a refusal of the medical professionals and/or facility to diagnose the pregnancy due to mainly an absence of the medically "appropriate" amount of HCG in a woman's blood. Defensive medicine is characterized by the fact that if anything should go awry and a medical professional and/or a medical facility were to be subjected to litigation, or simply a loss of "credibility," the medical professional has a better chance of protecting their interests.

In some cases I have come across, a pregnancy may be spotted and recorded in the medical records, but because of the practice of defensive medicine, the medical professionals themselves will refuse to attend to the woman as if she is pregnant.

"Extended Gestation," is any gestation that goes beyond the medical parameter of gestation, which is 42 weeks. While "Cryptic Pregnancy" (such as the pregnancies seen on "I Didn't Know I was Pregnant,") can not know how long the gestation went on for, before diagnosis or birth, CP/EG is more often than not, known to the mother about when conception exactly, or approximately took place. Often, CP/EGs extend up to 12 or 18 months and beyond.

In the many years since I had my CP/EG's and have been working with women experiencing CP/EG's, I have seen even medically documented pregnancies go up to about 18 months.

Approximately 1 in 450 women experience at least what is known medically as a "cryptic pregnancy." Some of these women are not aware that they are pregnant for part of the pregnancy or even the entire pregnancy. Some women are very aware of their cryptic pregnancy from the beginning. I was one of the latter women, twice. My first CP/EG baby was "cryptic" for the first three months and partly "cryptic" for the rest of the pregnancy. I gave birth to her at 44+ weeks in May of 2014. My second CP/EG baby was "cryptic" for at least five months and partly "cryptic" for the rest of the pregnancy. I would find out later that she was spotted in a sonogram and recorded in the medical records, but I was not informed, and the medical professionals at the time staunchly refused to treat me as if I was pregnant. I gave birth to her in August of 2015 at 52+ weeks.

About Me

My name is Anshin Kelly. I am a wife, and a mother of five healthy children. I am the Founder of the first "Traditional Wilderness Midwifery and Medicine" Practice. I am an alternative, intuitive healer and a Traditional Midwife, and now in recent months, a uniquely, and personally appointed "ECPM" (Extended and Cryptic Pregnancy Midwife). All of my children were born naturally and four of them were freebirth or unassisted births. In which there was no medical professional or midwife at their births. My husband was solely present for three of them and for one of the births, a few family members were also present. All children were healthy at birth and beyond. I have successfully breastfed all five of my children and did most of my own prenatal care for all five pregnancies.

I have been practicing alternative and energy medicine for fifteen years. I began my journey in the birth arts ten years ago when I became pregnant with my first baby. In those years I have worked with three incredible midwives in a patient as well as mentorship capacity, and now hundreds of women from all over the world; in person, online, over the phone and video chat, on their birth journeys.

In the time since my first CP/EG I have accumulated knowledge and experience in this realm through my hands on and consulting work. My learning and practice in this and all areas of health and birth are never done, but I have felt ready to in recent years, in an intuitive and practical way, expand my care of women and CP/EG with what I have deeply learned, observed, and experienced directly.

Section One: What Causes CP/EG?

CP/EG is, from what I've seen, almost completely denied and neglected by the medical field. As a result, CP/EG only has one very narrow definition; that from a Traditional Midwifery and Medicinal perspective, in my opinion, only serves to deny women's innate instinct. The only type of CP/EG that the medical field minimally recognizes is the kind in which a woman has either denial of the pregnancy, or blocked it out psychologically, and does not find out about her pregnancy until months into the pregnancy. In rarer cases, not until labor. Although I have seen medically documented cases of pregnancies extending up to 18 months, some women experiencing CP/EG symptoms sometimes report having so for years; and I have also, in recent years, observed real, flesh and blood babies, grow so slowly in the womb, their gestations span several years: Also in countries on the African Continent, such as Nigeria for example; CP/EG is more readily accepted by both Traditional and Medical Medicine alike. Women online, experiencing CP/EG in Nigeria, report that up to three years gestation is considered "normal" for women going through this already unique, and less common pregnancy experience.

The following is the result of my many years experience with CP/EG, and Traditional Healing and Birth Arts, as well as personal/collaborative research on the history of pregnancy, women's health and biology.

Communicating with the Medical Field

Communication with the medical field in my very intimate experience, especially with the subjects of pregnancy, natural birth, and CP/EG is exceptionally challenging. Why is it exceptionally challenging? I feel the main reasons are the following:

There seems to be coming from the very guts and roots of the educational systems and cultivation of medical professionals, not only a commitment to thorough medical training, but also a thorough commitment to cultivating a mentality of having reached a level of "expertise" that surpasses even a person's right to sense their own well-being and body; even to the extent that there is a "right" in the medical professional, to ignore a person's individual First Amendment Rights, in the name of "doing what is best, " for the patient. In other words; a mentality that says formal education itself gives one the power of *complete sight* and understanding of another individual. Even in the inherently mysterious and messy realm of scientific discovery, this goes against the fundamentals and principles of even Western Scientific research and discovery over the last 500 years. As well as, again, the fundamentals of bedrock America Freedoms and Principles. Madame Curie, I think, would be no less than horrified at some of the behaviors and mentalities I, and so many women have experienced, of our medical-modern-age. She gave her life, an ultimate act of sacrifice and humility for the sake of furthering human understanding of the Universe. Indeed humility is something that I feel our modern culture at large has mostly left to the wayside.

In my lifetime of experience, the majority of nursing assistants/ MD/OBGYN I've come into contact with seem to not be able to fathom that a person without their level of formal education could be more informed about their own mortal existence than them.

This I feel is at the root cause of why the deeply Intuitive, complex and mysterious realm of women's fertility and motherhood constantly bewilders, and even I feel at a fundamental level, frightens the collective beliefs and perspectives of the medical field.

Secondly, the medical field has become much too interested in its highly profitable role in modern society. This is NOT to say that even the majority of medical professionals are practicing simply for financial self-interests. However, the majority of people I have met throughout my life, who are studying to become anywhere from nursing assistants to MD's, have openly, and unabashedly admitted that one of the main reasons they are studying in their chosen medical field of study is to make a lot of money. Is there anything fundamentally wrong with wanting to make a lot of money? I don't happen to think so. But I do happen to think that making this a main reason one goes into a field of study that involves a most critically intimate access to human being's psyches, bodies and sense of well-being, is, fundamentally, and ethically unsound. This kind of motivation, in my experience, creates a psychological vulnerability in the budding medical professional, that potentially breeds mentalities that are divorced from our fundamental human instincts, about one's own mortal existence. In my experience, it seems to breed a sense of helplessness in the medical student/professional. What do I mean by a sense of helplessness? If a medical student/professional isn't fundamentally motivated by a pure desire to understand and help human beings and their health, then the mysteries and inherent challenges of assisting to heal and care for human beings will be crippling in their daunting affect. This seems to breed a need to maintain a sense of control and know-it-all, at all times, in the medical professional culture, and only serves to limit their ability to help people. Indeed I've heard medical students speak of the pressure they feel to "have all the answers". While I feel that pressure is certainly brought on by patients, I also feel that much of that pressure is brought on from an internal source as well, within the cultural structures of modern medical mentalities.

Addressing the Subject of Mental Illness

Understandably, many times the first thing that jumps into most people's heads when encountering the CP/EG experience is the subject of "phantom pregnancy" and/or mental illness.

Because the nature of CP/EG is that medical means of diagnosis tend to be insufficient, easily determining a case of "phantom" pregnancy or CP/EG is many times not simple. I use applied kinesiology as my main testing tool along with careful examination and observation of a woman's symptoms and I have found that more times than not, pregnancy symptoms start originally from just that, pregnancy. However, as I explain in the following sections, the CP/EG woman's endocrine and reproductive systems tend to have suffered past and/or current stress as well as trauma, and the slow and/or insufficient and/or dysfunctional release of hormones, as well as scarring and/or damage, tend to help create the CP/EG experience.

As mentioned before, I've worked with hundreds of women in their CP/EG experiences. Although there are some that seem to be either deeply scarred from life, CP/EG experiences, or cases of mental illness, the vast majority are not mentally ill and are simply experiencing a widely unknown and deeply misunderstood phenomenon with their bodies, hormones and pregnancies. This however can, as I explain in the following section, can lead to cases that land on a "spectrum" of instability for CP/EG mothers.

Mental and Emotional Vulnerability, and Instability in the CP/EG Woman

In my intimate experience with especially, and specifically North American Women and particularly CP/EG; I have learned the hard way that the Modern Woman is too often, extremely attached, even to the point of severe instability, to her *sense of control.* To be sure, being thrown into a situation such as CP/EG can cause even the most stable of women to reel; however, a cultural cultivation, and phenomenon in the Modern West, has caused women to deeply identify with their sense of control; that masquerades as being "empowered." It is a deep confusion; planted and cultivated for decades in the Modern West, between "being empowered," versus "having power."

This deeply entrenched sense of control, and cultural confusion; when suddenly confronted with a terribly misunderstood phenomenon such as CP/EG, will become extremely aggravated, challenged, and magnified. I have been at the wrong end of accusations, slander, ridicule, extreme disrespect, and cruel behavior, from overall, mostly the women themselves! The very women I have given the greater part of my emotional, physical, financial, and professional time and resources to; and to add to the massive disturbing mystery of this source of this abuse, *I am often the only one willing, and even able, to help them.*

Often, CP/EG women have lost their spouse's support, and even physical relationship. For a time, I attributed this mostly to the fact that their spouse and father of their CP/EG child could not accept the unique, and even taboo situation their wife and child are in; however, over time, I began to realize that the women themselves have been in a dysfunctional relationship themselves, to themselves, and therefore their spouse and loved ones, far before their CP/EG came about. Suddenly, not only can they not control their CP/EG, but they can not "convince" (or control) their spouse through their usual emotional routes, in their relationship dynamic. Desperate to maintain that sense of control they are accustomed to; their now aggravated sense of control tries to in a (sometimes extreme way), hold me hostage! They feel held hostage by their pregnancy situation, and to cope, they attempt to "hold me" emotionally "responsible," for their pregnancies, and yet, they (almost) never enter into a full Midwife/Patient "contract" with me. They keep their emotional (and physical) distance, while keeping themselves the "focal point" of their own lives (and attempting to make themselves the "victim" in mine). I feel one of the main reasons for this is because entrusting themselves to "the likes of me" (Anshin) would be "admitting" a loss of power, and control. At least a "genuine" doctor's inaccurate prognosis/diagnosis remains within their perceived sense of control; a doctor is "legitimate," while a Traditional Midwife is often, at the very least, controversial; and their perceived sense of control - for all (many) of their platitudes and outward attitudes about "independence" and "empowerment"- is hinged on *what other people think.*

I truly believe that CP/EG's are often more healthy, and come to term (whenever "term" means for the longer gestations), in places in Africa and Asia for example, because women in Africa and Asia are overall, rooted in cultural heritage that is thousands of years old. This cultural "Root System," lends itself to a natural, and cohesive *trust* in a Higher Power. In other words, the understanding that the Essence of Life itself can not ever be fully explained, or controlled, is inherent in thousands of generations of cultural, and spiritual continuity. Traditional Midwifery and

Medicine therefore, are more deeply woven, and therefore trusted within the historical fabric of a people.

Addressing Lying, Shame and Attention Seeking

The realm of CP/EG, especially in the modernized world, all over the world, is chaotic at this time. In my experience, one of the greatest wounds that a woman is faced with in her psyche is that of excessive shame. A healthy amount of shame in the psyche keeps us self-aware, but too many times the case is, since the beginning of time, that shame is used as an instrument of torture (also used by women) to keep a woman from knowing and seeking her power that is her birth-right.

Unfortunately, at this time, the more fanatical voices either "for" or "against" CP/EG are the loudest and many of us, who are striving to be the more reasonable, discerning and intuitive voices on the subject, tend to get painted with the same brush and/or drown out altogether- or as I've discovered in recent years, apparently stolen from.

It is in my experience, that at the core of this chaos is women's shame. In my chronic and extensive experience, the denial of our instincts and therefore on different levels, our humanity, invokes a deep and powerful shame that can send signals of frustration, to downright panic and/or even psychological shut-down in a woman. Being denied our feelings about our own bodies and so many times being written off as delusional and treated as if we have zero intelligence, by the medical field, and many times our family and friends, I have seen and experienced having a devastating effect on a woman's emotional, psychological and physical life. I have seen the despair women face send many of them into an obsessive and sometimes fanatical state about their CP/EG experience, as in, "for" or "against" the phenomenon. The CP/EG realm is often saturated in a chaotic and disparaging soup of extremes.

Some women even lie to cover up the shame they feel about insisting they feel pregnant, and then their body not continuing the pregnancy, and they are left feeling completely alone and abandoned and humiliated. Some deal with the shame and loneliness through incessant attention-seeking on social media about their CP/EG symptoms. Once in a while, a lonely or trolling woman or group of women will pretend to have CP/EG symptoms to be able to get into the facebook groups and actively spread toxicity, or simply be able to converse with others online as a way to pass the time.

One of the most devastating experiences I faced during my very early days with working in the CP/EG realm (I had already had both my CP/EG babies born in 2014 and 2015), which also almost pushed me to quit this work, was when a very young, very alone and desperate mother contacted me about her CP/EG. She also posted a video of her baby clearly kicking and moving inside her womb. If I remember correctly, not only were her instincts and her baby denied existence by the medical field, but she was prescribed a strong medication that she shared with me was not safe for pregnancy. She took it anyway, desperate to get rid of these "symptoms."

I was in correspondence with her for a few months. I believe it was a week or so after we last spoke on Facebook Messenger, that her family shared on Facebook their devastation at her taking her own life, leaving her two small children and husband behind. It took me many years to process the grief of this experience even this far, and part of that grief has been a deep anger towards the medical field and its chronic denial of these baby's lives and therefore their mother's lives. Now, to make matters worse, as soon as my work gains some traction, the same medical realm steals from me, and commodicizes these babies and mother's experiences. I am only able to write about it now, without bitterness, because I made the difficult decision years ago to keep on with this work, and eventually, educate the medical field and raise greater and greater awareness. I harbor minimal hard feelings. I just want better lives for these mothers and their babies, as well to heal, educate and open the realm of women's health at large, making greater space for the intuitive feminine, and sanctity of human life.

The bottom line I've come to find in this work, is that when it comes to CP/EG, women going through the phenomenon have been called to a very deep work; to be sure, we face some of our greatest fears and complexes in the process. This seems to be the nature of the experience and the work.

Section Two: Defensive Medicine

Beginning with my own situation, many "cryptic" pregnancy cases boil down to the simple and troubling fact that a medical professional/institution simply refuses to diagnose and/or treat a woman as if she is pregnant because of the "too low" or lack of HCG in the pregnant woman's blood. A baby in these cases IS spotted on the sonogram and/or fetal tones are officially documented but denied existence simply because of the lack of HCG. These cases seem to be extensively treated by the medical field as a professional liability. Acting in this way, to put the legal and professional interests before a patient's well-being, is known as "defensive medicine". In my opinion, defensive medicine is a plague on the health realm at large.

Recently, I found that Healthline.com published in their article on cryptic pregnancy, that a fetus could be missed in a sonogram due to the fact that it is positioned in the uterus "irregularly." This article was published on February 26th, 2019. Besides the fact that I, and hundreds of other women who have had intimacy with CP/EG could testify to the fact that even three years ago, the only information regarding CP/EG on the internet on mainstream sites, were essentially what these sources and journalists mined from the hit show "I Didn't Know I Was Pregnant;" I published many, many videos on the subject of ultrasound inaccuracy because of things such as unexpected uterine and fetal positioning, between 2018 and 2019. Indeed my own story regarding my second CP/EG is centered in large part around this fact.

In a particular case I worked with the mother's medical records state that they had seen on the sonogram a full-term pregnancy (anywhere from a four pound and higher baby) at some point during the visit, but never told her. She continued through the entire experience without any prenatal care, support, or guidance. When she got in touch with me I offered to do a form of testing called "muscle testing" or "applied kinesiology." I picked up that she had conceived three times in the two years that she has been pregnant; and that two were no longer viable and one was still alive. She later sent her sonogram photos to a Doctor in Africa named "Dr. Impo" (his online work can be found at impocity.blogspot.com) who had written back that there were two masses above and below the viable fetus in her womb. We both felt that this had confirmed my testing.

At one point towards the end of her CP/EG a head nurse from the hospital diagnosed her pregnancy via doppler, but the OB/GYN refused to see her; we could only assume this was because of the lack of HCG from her first few visits at the beginning of her pregnancy.

She didn't get in touch for two years after that. When she finally wrote to me she said that I had been right about my intuitions about the woman's body in many cases reabsorbing the pregnancies, (see section below; "missed miscarriage"). She shared she had been experiencing heavy hemorrhaging and blood clots, but her body was in the process of going back to normal.

Section Three: The Endocrine System of the CP/EG Woman, and Female Reproductive Medicalization

As mentioned before, I use applied kinesiology as my main form of testing in my work. During all my pregnancies including and especially my CP/EG's I developed muscle testing specifically for pregnancy and childbirth. It is through this vehicle as well as on-going experience, hands-on work and research that I came to understand more fully the endocrine system of the CP/EG woman.

Women going through CP/EG seem to have one very consistent thing in common: Their endocrine systems have suffered under severe stress/trauma, and/or their overall reproductive health has been heavily medicalized. The causes of this trauma and medicalization seem to be consistently aligned with one or more of the following:

- Multiple Pregnancies close together

- Breastfeeding
- Weight Issues
- History of medically diagnosed glandular dysfunction
- Multiple reproductive/or other surgeries
- Chemotherapy/Other forms of medical/invasive cancer treatment
- Sexual Trauma
- Abusive/Dysfunctional Relationships
- Any/All forms of hormonal birth control
- Abortion(s)
- Miscarriage(s)
- Cesarean Section(s)
- Epidural(s)
- Plan-B taken one or more times
- Poor/highly processed diet, drinking and/or drugs and general bodily neglect and/or ignorance

In my experience, the CP/EG woman's endocrine system and overall reproductive system, can be anywhere from too stressed to downright despondent. Everything in between seems to be a possibility.

Recently I discovered that Healthline.com in the same article mentioned above, artfully concealed in an "anecdotal common sense" tone, wrote that there is a connection between being very young and pregnant, and the confusion and/or complications that arise from the CP/EG experience. In January 22nd, 2019 I published a YouTube video entitled *"The Truth About the Cryptic Pregnancy Community,"* where I mention, as a pivotal factor in the confusion and mystery surrounding CP/EG experience, that; *"My sense about many very young women going through this experience, is that they are just simply not informed and/or educated properly about basic, reproductive biology."* In my intimate, heartfelt, and grounded experience with CP/EG, no one has cared enough to make any sort of helpful connection or discovery anywhere for these women and their babies, let alone something as specific, or even close to as observational as that. In fact, young women are routinely prescribed reproductive medications, and/or pressured into invasive reproductive procedures such as abortion; that in my intimate experience and observation seemed to have led them to the experience of CP/EG.

Similar mainstream sites are also consistently listing the connection between birth control and CP/EG, and are dated around the time most of my CP/EG videos came out, as well as the first preliminary publication of my CP/EG Ebook guide. Again, in all the years I've been in the trenches with these women and babies, the constant, tragic and frustrating reality has been that many of these women have been on medications, and/or subjected to heavy medications and major surgeries regarding their reproductive health over the course of a sometimes many decades. However, the same medical professionals that prescribed and carried out these medical decisions, will routinely turn around and flatly deny their longtime female patient's CP/EG symptoms. Even, in some extreme cases, diagnose them as in need of psychological treatment, and additional medicating.

One of the first women I assisted during her CP/EG said that, "The same doctor who delivered my multiple children now denies my CP/EG. Back when my now, grown children were in utero, ultrasound testing was not mainstream yet, and extended gestation was more readily regarded as normal. When my lab tests came back negative, my male doctor stated, *'Well, it walks like a duck and quacks like a duck, so it must be a duck.'* He proceeded to treat those pregnancies with no trouble, and my children were delivered under his care, also with no trouble."

From what I remember, this woman's doctor flatly denied this woman's CP/EG for over a year at least, and indeed denied her care overall. Without any explanation one day, he promptly prescribed her a hysterectomy procedure, after a series of tests she finally convinced him to do.

I have heard and read many stories of CP/EG babies discovered during CP/EG mother's various surgical reproductive procedures, and once in a very great while I will come across stories of babies that don't survive the procedures. Unfortunately, I'll come across more stories in my work than I think most people would be able to face, where I deeply suspect that a doctor will decide to abort a CP/EG baby under the pretense of other reproductive medical reasoning. The mother's story above, is just one example of my heartbreaking sense, in this regard.

Section Four: Positioning of the Uterus

Websites such as the ones mentioned above, I've discovered also are beginning to casually mention that placement, and shape of the uterus may also play a role in negative sonogram results. Again, I can testify to the fact that the very idea of something like the positioning or shape of a woman's uterus could be a factor in CP/EG, and negative ultrasound, was not only widely ridiculed and/or at the very least dismissed by the medical field, and the internet realms at large; but mainstream pop- journalism-centric medical sites, would never dream of hinting at such a thing. I am the only one I know of who has produced extensive information regarding the subject. Indeed, I was interviewed for over an hour by a producer of the daytime TV show "Dr. Phil," four years ago, as if she were doing a documentary rather than an episode of the drama/reality-based series that Dr. Phil is. I could tell she really wanted me on the show, however, the person they ended up bringing on I know for a fact is a fanatic "against" CP/EG, and has personally slandered me on multiple occasions on her YouTube channel. I eventually ended up producing proof that this YouTube personality was lying about her presumed medical credentials; and I presented this proof to her nursing school director, as well as the nursing board she would presumably be affiliated with.

In other words, the focus even four years ago when it came to CP/ EG for major forums and platforms at large, was drama, and a "let's harass and/or have a slice of the freak-show that is CP/EG," kind of agenda, and feel.

I continued to be the only one I know of, with anything to say at all about CP/EG that is experienced based, thoroughly researched and in-depth, even at the height of the social CP/EG "freak-show" era. Now it seems, the tide is turning, but I maintain with unwavering conviction that there must be accountability and proper acknowledgement of the pioneers of the CP/EG realm.

A very common condition of the CP/EG woman is having a retroverted uterus. I have also seen in sonogram photos what clearly looks like a uterus with either a full or partial septum. Creating two basic compartments. Insights from other women and myself describe it as the baby being tucked away in the back, causing sometimes a great amount of pressure and discomfort in the lower back and hips.

Studying sonogram photos and medical reports of women's abdomens, as well as practicing vaginal and abdominal exams myself for CP/EG mothers (including myself) has led me to the conclusion that due to past or present stress and/or trauma women's bodies, like many mammals, will tuck the pregnancy way back towards the spine. Their organs will become positioned in front of the uterus to protect the growing fetus.

Section Five: Scarring of the Uterus and Glandular System

Uterine scarring is very common in the modern age. The loose and expedient performing of invasive procedures and their traumatic effect on a woman's body, glaringly make themselves known in the making of a CP/EG situation. Over the years in my experience, these procedures and medications include any and/or multiple of the following: Cesarean sections, abortions and/or other invasive surgical procedures in which the woman is put under heavy medications that deeply affect her natural cycle; such as plan-b and all forms of hormonal birth control.

This scarring of the uterus and glandular system I have seen over and over again, contribute to the making of a CP/EG situation. This includes both the making of "negative" lab tests as well as unclear or "negative" sonograms.

PART TWO

What Causes Extended Gestation and Symptoms?

Delayed Development of a fetus is a phenomenon that the Western Scientific community has only somewhat researched and observed in mammals. I certainly have witnessed it first hand growing up on a farm, and then in my two CP/EG's. I have also suspected and/or witnessed it in several pregnancies that are not considered CP/EG.

This phenomenon is definitely connected to stress. This stress can be anywhere between medium-consistent stress and a severe amount of stress.

Another casual, anecdotal "connection" to CP/EG the the medial-pop-journalists are now making in the last few years, is its relationship to stress and neglect. Since 2016 I have been making videos and putting out post after post, not to mention my ebooks on the subject in the last four years, about the connection to stress, neglect, lack of community and regard for womanly intuition, that CP/EG has.

My first ebook I published four years ago, is an herbal guide for CP/EG and the first of its kind. I have also put out videos about my extensive observation and personal experience regarding the essential role that herbalism and nutrition has in relation to CP/EG. Some of those sources I have go as far back as 2018, which is also when I began to see the change and alleged plagiarism in mainstream medical sites. It seems medical-pop-journalists have farmed these ideas from me as well, and per usual evasion of accountability in citing sources, have cloaked these insights and mentions in "anecdotal common sense."

Well, I continue to maintain, if this is so common sense, then where is the medical option for CP/EG women in pretty much any hospital anywhere in North America? I am quite sure if there was any such thing, I would have heard of it by now.

One of the stories of delayed development that stands out in my work, is the following:

A homosexual woman received medical fertilization to get pregnant. She began having classic CP/EG symptoms in which her body was shifting and changing for apparent pregnancy, but could not be medically diagnosed. She continued having these symptoms for three years. When she finally became medically confirmed, because of the rising amount of HCG in her system, the medical professionals were persistent and thorough with her sonogram procedures and they were eventually able to find a fetus measuring eleven weeks. From what I understand, it was difficult even then in the process to find the fetus in ultrasound. I'd also like to add here that it's pretty common among CP/EG women to have had one or more non-CP/EG pregnancies that were difficult to spot in a sonogram, detect in a lab as well as difficult for them to feel in the uterus from the inside. Their CP/EG's then seem to be just an exaggerated version of what they have already experienced.

I have also been able to have hands-on, consistent experience and observation with women whose CP/EG experiences have lasted 2-4+ (give or take) years, but have excellent health. This is less common than most experiencing healthy CP/EG's, as most will give birth naturally, be medically confirmed, induced or given a c-section, or miscarry after carrying for 17-18 months or less. Most of the women I have encountered and worked with whose CP/EG experiences are lasting years, have current, many times severe health issues that they refuse to address. They tend to ignore possible signs of miscarriage during those years, and unfortunately seem very content to be trapped where they are.

However, healthy women whose experiences last sometimes 2-4+ years and whose pregnancies seem healthy, seem to be experiencing long delays in development during that time period. With careful months of observation and in-depth explanations of their symptoms and experiences, I deeply suspect that long delays in development that last months, even years occur especially in the very early stages of development. As mentioned before this is sometimes seen in the mammal world, for example: Sometimes female bears will mate right before hibernation, and the conception will be incubated/paused. Her body will then proceed with implantation and the continued growth of the baby come spring. I suspect this "incubation/preservation" process that a woman's body instigates in times of stress (including the many times invasive procedures involved in artificial insemination) would explain a lot when it comes to the CP/EG phenomenon in women.

One of the first things that I noticed when it came to mainstream medical sources in regards to farming my work, was the casual mention that, "cryptic pregnancy may last longer than usual pregnancies." One site recently went so far as to add that, "there isn't any credible research in regards to the length of cryptic pregnancy," and yet bothered to mention that there is some speculation on that matter. Speculation? On what basis? From whom?

One third of women in America are given cesarean sections, many times on the premise that their baby "is overdue and might die." Around forty-one percent of women are induced, also on the premise that their baby is "overdue." So I ask again, speculation that specifically CP babies might gestate longer in the womb? On what basis? Medical culture is generally hell-bent on removing the child from their mother's supposedly "risk-filled" body!

Another thing that these sites seem to be mentioning in the same breath is that there is evidence that CP babies seem to often come out "premature." So again, where is this "speculation" about CP babies having longer gestations coming from? I am confident that I am most likely the sole "expert" on the subject in North America, and the only one not only sharing about the evidence that extended gestation exists, but can share with extensive knowledge from hands-on experience, on the subject.

Section One: A CP/EG Mother's Physical Reaction to Her Pregnancy

Recently, I described to a CP/EG mother in an analogy, what her body was going through, and why her body and baby were supporting, and growing in the way that they are. I said:

"The vast majority of CP/EG mothers have been through some kind of physical, medical and/or emotional trauma prior and/or during their CP/EG. You can imagine your body is like your house. You have everything set up the way you like and expect. Maybe when you bought the house there were major repairs needed, and you were able to come up with the money, energy and other resources to make that happen. Maybe after you bought the house, one time, some kid threw a baseball and broke your window, and another time a branch fell in a storm and brought the electrical lines down that go to your house. Again, you were able to gather the resources to repair all of these mishaps and damages...

You and your husband are faring well, even though the financial and energy strain, due to the damages and repairs, have at times taken a toll...then, a family member walks in, needing a place to stay. You can't turn them away, and nor do you want to, however, your house, and relationship dynamics in relation to your house, was not fully developed or equipped for this family member's sudden residence. Suddenly, you can not get up in the middle of the night and watch TV on the couch, because your guest is sleeping there! Suddenly, if you and your husband are having an argument, you can't just let it rip wherever you want to in the house! Things have to adjust, but in order for everything to not snap under the strain of the new dynamic- you must take things more slowly, more measuredly. Suddenly, certain major avenues in life, like: Finances, emotions, habits etc. must slow down, in order to accommodate to the new, sudden change in dynamic."

I said to the mother also: "You are healing while growing a baby. This is the CP/EG process."

A CP/EG woman's body is reacting to the major event, of the conception of the child; whose relationship to her is as deeply personal as it is "foreign," in an extreme way. Much like the reaction a household might have to the sudden appearance, and dependency of a guest, the body must now take a very measured stock of everything within its own, intimate and metabolic dynamic. In order to keep both the mother and baby as safe as possible, the mother's body establishes a *"Hibernation-Adaptation Pattern,"* that allows for the distribution of resources for growth and healing, in a way that prevents the entire "household" from collapsing. This wisdom of the mother's body, and her baby, I have come to understand, and experience as totally astounding, and miraculous.

Section Two: Getting Pregnant While Pregnant

Although human history has been far from perfect, there was a consistent level of consciousness throughout ancient societies that acknowledged and accepted the deep, mysterious quality and aspect of Life itself. Western science, in my years of research and experience, does acknowledge the reality of "superfetation", or getting pregnant while pregnant. But like so many biological phenomena in the female human and mammalian world, it is hardly touched on in easily accessible material, let alone considered a possibility to look into. Especially when unusual situations such as CP/EG symptoms occur.

The deeply mysterious and hidden parts of life include those phenomena that we are not, in many instances, there to look at under a microscope. I feel that superfetation is one of these phenomena. Some medical data is recorded that concludes outwardly that it does in fact occur. Although the vast majority of times it occurs it's either simply because women are unaware that it is happening (i.e the second conception can not sustain itself because the first one takes precedence in the body) or because the only way to know is through the woman herself applying intuition and self-knowledge. The realm of Western medicine in my, and so many other women's experiences does not seem to put any significant value in this kind of deep self-care and knowing. The "lay-man-over-expert" model of practice seems to be foundational to medical practice.

In many cases of CP/EG, I have suspected through applied kinesiology, raw experience and intuition that superfetation plays a role.

Another subject that pop-medical-journalism is now mentioning "anecdotally" is the connection between getting pregnant very soon after birth and CP. Americanpregnancy.com, although does not mention the date of publication, makes this "casual-common sense" claim in their article on cryptic pregnancy. I have spoken about this pattern of pregnancy- right- after-birth, in CP/EG women including with my own CP/EG experiences since as far back as 2015. But the preliminary release of my ebook was 2020, and I officially include it there as part of my extensive and intimate experience and observational data on CP/EG.

Section Three: Missed Miscarriage

Over the years I have seen medically documented reports of a mother's body being able to reabsorb a miscarry. This is also a biological response that can commonly be seen in rabbits and other mammals when they experience deficiencies. A litter/baby animal is simply reabsorbed into the body and the body expels blood clots. This can happen even with a human baby of substantial size; anywhere from four pounds and higher:

This may seem unbelievable for many, or even most; but it's extremely important to understand firstly, that a baby's "bones" even at birth, are largely made up of cartilage. It is equally unbelievable for most that a woman experiencing a cryptic pregnancy, could be unaware that she is pregnant, but it happens!

The larger the baby is, in the event of "reabsorption," the more hemorrhaging occurs. In humans, this type of miscarriage is often called a "missed miscarriage" or a "silent miscarriage."

In many cases of women who feel they have been pregnant with the same baby for multiple years (claims of 2-7 years are commonly seen), it is common to see mild to severe health issues present in addition to the CP/E experience.

With one of my first experiences regarding the reabsorption and breaking down of a good sized baby, the mother was in a state of dissonance. She knew instinctively that she was pregnant. She also had all the obvious signs of pregnancy, including a baby belly and movement. However, she was so distraught and conflicted about being pregnant that she would party and drink regularly. She had pregnancy symptoms for one year, messaging and sending me pictures and videos regularly.

One day, I muscle tested her baby's health and it was obvious the baby wasn't going to make it. Shortly after she began hemorrhaging heavily, passing huge blood clots daily. I gave her suggestions and dosages for herbal remedies to help slow the bleeding. If my memory is correct, I don't believe she ever took the herbs. However, the bleeding continued in this heavy way for a month, so she finally made an appointment with her doctor and was prescribed birth control pills. The pill did help to control the bleeding.

She didn't message me for around a year after that. When she finally did her body had gone back to normal and she informed me that she felt that the whole thing had been psychological. I will admit I was heartbroken that a woman would deny and bury her experience so severely. The lack of support, neglect, and even downright abuse causes many women in similar experiences to reject their intuitive experiences with their own bodies. As well as barely acknowledge my work and investment in assisting them on and through their journeys.

As said before, phenomena such as superfetation and delayed development are not only rooted in biological responses to stress and trauma-related conditions, but are in my experience also rooted in the psychological, emotional, and spiritual realities that are at the root cause of why a mother's body feels it must protect a pregnancy to such a large extent. Including her baby also feeling the need to adapt to detected stress/trauma/danger in this way; causing what is known as CP/EG.

Having said that, the vast majority of CP/EG's in North America, and in the generally developed, medicalized West, will end in miscarriage. The main reason for this I feel, is because women are deeply influenced and conditioned in the West, by not only the systemic medicalization of their bodies; but are also generationally indoctrinated in ideas about "empowerment" that have only led to widespread isolation, and a growing issue of societal depression, loneliness; and therefore a growing dependence on medications to try and stem the psychological hemorrhage of the *inner reality* of disempowerment.

I would like to add here that in my experience, as well as many other women's experiences that I know of, a woman's body is seen by the medical field as mainly mechanical in nature, rather than fundamentally mysterious, powerful and intuitive in nature. Although the idea that a woman's body can reabsorb a baby, and dispel blood clots, even with a baby of a good size, can be challenging at first to understand and imagine; after seeing pattern after pattern, of women, obviously pregnant, even medically diagnosed in their medical records, miscarry this way, and then return to a non-pregnant state; I knew I had to go deeper, when it came to my current understanding.

I'm going to leave this for now as food-for-thought, as well as for body and soul:

If a woman's body could make every last microscopic cell of that child's body, then her body certainly has the innate intelligence to reclaim, and breakdown every last cell, as well.

Section Four: Bleeding While Pregnant

Another "anecdotal-common-sense" mention I have found more and more in pop-medical-journalism, is the never-before-now, mentioned reality of continued bleeding while pregnant. If it were "common knowledge," as well as a topic of medical discussion, I wouldn't have suffered the way I did, as I will now explain in the following:

I became aware of the phenomenon of bleeding while pregnant when I was pregnant with my first baby, who was not a CP/EG. She was however always difficult to spot in a sonogram. Even at a pretty good size. To my horror and extreme anxiety, I began bleeding at around four months gestation. I was not aware at all that it was possible to bleed while having a healthy pregnancy. Instinctively, I knew the baby was ok, but I was conditioned like most Western women to only associate bleeding during pregnancy with death and miscarriage.

I bled for ten days straight, sometimes heavily, and every color it seemed on the blood-red spectrum. I finally made an appointment to get an ultrasound and the result was what I instinctively already knew; the baby was healthy and literally kicking- but still evasive, and a challenge to see clearly in ultrasound.

The bleeding eventually stopped shortly after that, and I went on to have a very healthy pregnancy and natural birth.

I would bleed during pregnancy for the rest of my children. Resulting in healthy, natural, unassisted births of four healthy girls and one boy.

Bleeding while pregnant is extraordinarily common in CP/EG. Like so many symptoms in relation to CP/EG in my observation and experience, bleeding while pregnant is mainly caused by the following:

- Insufficient hormone excretion
- Chronic/everyday to severe stress
- Past and/or current trauma and PTSD due to sexual, emotional, verbal, mental, and other physical abuse.
- Extended or/short term use of hormonal birth control, and invasive medical procedures such as C-sections, abortions, and other surgeries.
- A history of difficult/stressful menstrual cycles and/or pregnancies
- Nutritional deficiency
- Indiscriminate sexual lifestyles often combined with:
- Substance Abuse- such as alcohol.

Bleeding while pregnant seems to be heavily connected to the woman's body struggling to maintain a balanced production of progesterone. As many of you know, progesterone has two main purposes; to help build and maintain a healthy and thickened endometrial lining in preparation and/or event of a conception. As well as to prevent the over-production of estrogen; a counterbalance to prevent the hyper-growth of the endometrial lining. Its purpose is both to support growth as well as growth prevention. I feel that understanding more holistically, the nature of progesterone and its central role in assisting a woman's body in the natural ups and downs of her cycles and fertility, is one of the cornerstone keys to understanding and assisting in CP/EG.

Section Five: The Connection Between Death and Loss, and CP/EG

It became evident over the course of about seven years, and assisting hundreds of CP/EG women through various levels of their journeys; that it was more common than I originally realized, for CP/EG women to have experienced a loss in the past, of a child or a spouse. To begin with, I saw right away, through my own CP/EG's and very soon, while working with a few cases that; a woman experiencing the CP/EG phenomenon was coming directly into contact with a kind of phenomenal "Death in Life" shift within every layer and facet of her life. Seeing the way close friends, family, spouses, and health care providers would, over and over again, in various cases, react/respond to the CP/EG as if their friend/wife/patient were claiming she had three heads instead of one; was all at once disturbing, as well as fascinating to me. My immediate family and husband had been very supportive when particularly one of my CP/EG's was clearly proving to be out of the realm we were (and most) are used to. They, and I, could not understand why husbands were routinely refusing to speak about their wife's CP/EG experience, and/or even leaving their wife because of it. It is also common for the CP/EG woman's husband to then participate in third-party gossip, humiliation, and alienation of their former wife, and mother of their child.

It struck me that women who knew Death, in an intimate way, such as losing a child or a spouse- sometimes that loss was not physical death, but prison, or severe trauma of another kind- would often then be the ones among women who experience CP/EG. Somehow "Death," whether physical, or in another sense; such as abandonment or trauma is a central, indeed, a core theme that is set in motion, through the conception of a very unique new life within a CP/EG woman. Often, I wonder if the child conceived was meant to grow to term; or their central "mission" in a sense was to cause this cataclysmic shift inside the mother- and indeed the society around her.

Section Six: Inefficient, and Insufficient Water Absorption: Limited Accumulation

and Sustaining of Amniotic Fluid

The shape and size of the CP/EG mother's pregnant belly is, for the inexperienced person, at times, a bewildering reality to behold. The women who "Didn't Know I Was Pregnant," can testify greatly to this bewildering reality and phenomenon. Of course, as mentioned before, the positioning of the uterus is deeply connected to the inability for sonograms to find and diagnose a pregnancy; however, I have also discovered and concluded over the course of almost a decade, that the production, and maintaining of amniotic fluid in a CP/EG mother, is for some reason difficult. As a result, the mother's body and baby feel a very real lack of protection: The amniotic fluid serves many vital purposes in growing a baby, but its main role is protection of the baby, as well as the mother.

Like everything else in a CP/EG, the production and maintenance of amniotic fluid is being delayed, in order to prevent the body, and Being (the mother) from total collapse; both physically and psychologically. We are made up of mostly water, and so the inability for the mother's body to produce and maintain amniotic fluid means that there is a heightened to severe problem regarding water intake/absorption.

The CP/EG mother's belly will often remain soft outwardly, but she will feel the baby's mass tucked way back towards her spine, and nestled snugly in her hips. Fetal movement is often difficult for mothers to detect. The mother's belly will often also come out, especially when they report, during times the mother feels calm and safe, and the baby will also move a lot in these instances. However, the baby/belly will inevitably recede back inside the mother's body.

At about four years into working with many CP/EG cases, I began to be able to "measure" the health/progress of the pregnancy based on whether the baby/belly was, albeit slowly, becoming more predisposed to staying outward; and therefore the mother's belly remaining more firm (and full of amniotic fluid).

Section Seven: CP/EGs Extending Beyond 18 Months:

In the last four years or so, I have been able to observe very closely and consistently CP/EGs that extend beyond eighteen months. So far the longest CP/EG I have had consistent observations and appointments with, has lasted going on five years, and is currently in the preparatory labor stage.

As I've mentioned prior; in my experience over the last eight years with CP/EG, I have seen consistently that the vast majority of CP/EGs will resolve in some way between 12 and 18 months. This means that the women will have their baby (sometimes through surgical means and/or induction), or miscarry. To review; there are two types of miscarriages that I have witnessed many times in CP/EG women, and they are the following:

The first one is a regular miscarriage, in which the baby is expelled completely from the mother's body, and the second is called a missed miscarriage or silent miscarriage. In my experience, in the cases of missed miscarriage, the mother's body will either completely reabsorb a baby, or partially reabsorb the baby, and expel the rest.

There are, however, CP/EGs that do last longer than eighteen months. Some testimonies online have claimed having been pregnant for up to ten years. I do not so far have experience with this length of CP/EG, however, I can say the following:

Women who testify having experienced their CP/EG for up to ten years or more, in my experience, will either only claim this particular experience for themselves as a personal testimony, or some will make a case, without much proof beyond their own experience, that this kind of CP/EG is a possibility for women at large. Meaning, they either do not claim their testimony to be of a general, universal nature in women at large, or they will aggressively try and advocate their theories, without much foundation beyond personal testimonials, to women they have met online, and connected to on social media.

I personally feel that a CP/EG experience that is extending up to a decade, is a combination of physical, and spiritual imbalances, in a woman's sexual, and social life, as well as hormonal, mental, and spiritual health. For some reason, her central need for bringing forth life, and nurturing life as a woman, is in crisis, and needs comprehensive, hands-on healing.

The women who are experiencing CP/EGs for over 18 months, that I have been able to work with directly, all have one or more of the following in common:

Histories of physical/sexual, emotional, spiritual, reproductive or other trauma.

Histories of reproductive or other illness, and/or surgery

Histories of having taken subscription medicine, and/or are currently prescribed medication.

Complicated, strained, and/or abusive relationships with their baby's father.

A pattern that most share is that when they are at the 18th month to two year mark, their often very ambiguous, and/or slow-growing symptoms of pregnancy up until this point, will then begin growing more consistently, albeit slowly.

My first anchoring point for understanding what to look for in a CP/EG woman, in terms of health, and growth of their baby, was to look for consistent growth; it didn't matter if it was slowly, what mattered was that there was exponential, trackable growth, and no longer long periods of ambiguity, and dormancy.

I have seen and heard stories of women getting their CP/EGs medically confirmed finally, after experiencing pregnancy symptoms for over two years. From what I understand, and to my knowledge, the women went on to have healthy babies. The primary, and usually only reason to my knowledge that their pregnancy symptoms are finally taken seriously by the medical field, is that the HCG levels in their blood are finally elevated enough for the hospital to consider "positive."

Section Eight: Preparatory Labor Period: The Struggle to Give Birth; Relating to Modern Women's Psyche, and Bodies

The Preparatory Labor Period in a CP/EG can take many, many months, especially if the pregnancy has lasted two or more years.

In a CP/EG woman, there has been a "seizure," to varying levels, of and within her uterine, as well as overall reproductive function: This seizure is happening on at least two levels of being; psychological and physical. The word "seizure" also has a couple of meanings: One is to "capture" something or someone, and the other is a physiological condition, in which a person has what is known as "a seizure." In the second instance, a person having a seizure is experiencing a sudden attack, or convulsion, or spasms, usually relating to the heart or brain; which are both epi-centers within the body for relating messages and commands, for every facet of the body's function. This includes muscular and hormonal functions.

Psychologically, Western and/or Modern women at large are more often than not, in my lifetime of experience, "captured." What are they captured by, and why are they captured? Well, it is mostly, at its core, a *paralyzing sense of shame.*

Roughly, 1 in 5 women that I've befriended, and/or worked with, and/or have had as my client, have had some traumatic, and shameful, sexual experience before the age of 19. I can only guess, because of this psychological paralysis of roughly one-fifth of women predominantly up to the age of 40 or so, this tragic and rampant, current social reality is not discussed, almost ever. In fact, in my lifetime of experience, the *silence* as they say *is deafening*. I can also only ascertain through intimate observation, that one of the greatest reasons why the silence is deafening, is because the women themselves work very hard, first inside their own minds, and then in how they carry out their lives, to keep it that way:

Tragically, in the last thirty or so years, the accessibility of alcohol, drugs, and sexually explicit content, as well as social permissions for minors, have exploded to a degree in which our parents lost total control of the reins quite a long time ago. Now, us, their children are all in our late twenties, thirties, and early forties; and one of the central outfalls of the societal fabric of which we are made, is that: It is *"every 'liberated and independent ' woman for herself."*

To put it lightly - this is not conducive to the conception and birth of new life.

This goes back to the deeply entrenched confusion between "empowerment " versus "having power," and therefore identifying heavily with control.

Being "captured" sexually, especially from a young age, is extremely harmful and painful for anyone, but particularly for girls and women. When one considers the amount that women's bodies, especially surrounding reproduction have been medicalized and exploited in the modern age, the picture begins to come into focus regarding why "seizure" happens to a woman's womb, in reaction to a conception; creating what is known as "cryptic pregnancy" or what I've come to call "cryptic pregnancy and extended gestation (CP/EG)." This same paralysis I speak of in a woman's psyche, is echoing many times over, and expressing itself in large part, through the CP/EG phenomenon. The healing then, must be the process of "freeing" or "unseizing" the psyche and womb.

Miscarriage is vastly common, and birth rare in CP/EG and the (over)developed West because the ability to let go of control, and therefore allow "Life through Death," is being suffocated on a systemic level. As a CP/EG mother said to me once, "the uterus is constipated," indeed! And, she continued, "we need to figure out why the uterus is constipated."

Exactly.

In my deep experience, most women's bodies will miscarry and process a miscarriage all on its own, with little to no danger to the mother. However, there are instances I feel strongly, that a woman and her baby could die, if the mother has not, and can not truly awaken herself to her need to *let go*. Modern women, especially CP/ EG women, will spend a lot of time placing blame on others for their predicaments. They are often angry, and rightfully so, but seem to not be able to understand deeply enough that no matter what wrongs others have inflicted upon us;

our lives are ultimately our responsibility- and, there is a Higher Law and Love at work, all the time, that is completely out of our control. In other words, our only hope in seeing things through in life, whatever they are, is to relinquish our false sense of control, and trust in that Higher Law and Love; of and from whence our babies are totally made- and therefore ultimately we, ourselves, also.

PART THREE

More Stories, Experiences, and Wisdom, Reclaimed from Walking with CP/EG Babies and Mothers

CP/EG, more than anything in my experience, is an immeasurably deep reclamation, especially for Westernized women at large, of the Sacred Feminine. The womanly intuition was widely condemned through the Westernizing of the world, and fanatical Christian viewpoints, for hundreds of years. The ancient, sacred religious rites, traditions and motifs of the Goddess and the Sacred Feminine, were routinely desecrated, smashed, and overlaid with Christianized, male views on what a woman is, and who she must be on a personal, familial and societal level.

Here is a passage from a blog post I wrote in 2019:

"An Injured, Modern Complex and Behavior: More Unusual Womanly Experiences are Deservingly Subject to Neglect, Abuse and Ridicule

One can also trace the centrality of this concept in modern culture to "The Burning Times," and this beginning of the end of up to millions of years of continuity in Wise Women Traditions and Traditional Midwifery practices. The main reason for this being, the wiping out of a culturally driven and accepted need for woman to woman connection, community and culture; created by and for women. Women for thousands of years sought the shelter, healing and wisdom of the Village Wise Women and their community's woman network. Over the last few hundred years, beginning in Europe and Colonial America a now deeply rooted connection between wealth and societal status, and women giving up the natural womanly arts of breastfeeding, baby-wearing, and all around hands on care of their own children, lives on in our modern culture. Isolation is confused with independence and empowerment. Generally, women in modern culture compete for positions of power and popularity, "every woman for herself," much the way men do in patriarchal societies, rather than cultivating sisterhood, womanly support and networking."

Being a woman for many hundreds of years in the West, became an overall inferior existence. Westernized women today in my lifelong experience, do not generally help to introspectively analyze and find paths to healing this legacy of oppression, but in fact chronically buy into Westernized, injured male viewpoints and behavior concerning points of power, position and societal status.

Therefore, not only, on a collective psychological level are women considered inferior, even and in some cases especially by women, but an unusual woman is even more subject to abuse on many more levels of social structure than most.

In my many years experience and field-work in the realm of CP/ EG, I have come to understand on a deep level that the source of the problem lies in collective, Western conditioning, not in CP/EG itself. In most cases, CP/EG is, when observed carefully, patiently and intuitively over time, not the central issue. The central issues lie in how a woman is conditioned to see and treat herself, and how her family and/or society are conditioned to see and treat her. Additionally, more often than not, if a CP/EG is causing health issues for the woman, it is because of a terribly tangled mass of issues, viewpoints and decisions that were made, sometimes many years leading up to the CP/EG.

One such CP/EG stands out in my heart and mind concerning how, many medically-centered decisions are central to the making of a CP/EG that is causing sometimes severe issues for the woman's health and well-being:

A woman and her husband traveled many miles from out of state to have an in-person consultation with me. She had been experiencing a CP/EG for over a year at least. To say the least, the experience had been so difficult, and physically painful at times, the woman had shared with me that she had taken time to write her Last Will and Testament, because the pain she was experiencing sometimes was so, very severe.

This particular CP/EG was nothing that I'd really experienced or come across at that point, and I'd seen many, many very unusual things over the years. The woman had gotten a partial hysterectomy a few years prior, and when she conceived after the operation, it had been to say the least, one of the greatest shocks of her life. But she is a mother of multiple children, and she expressed to me that "The intuitive knowledge as a woman that you're pregnant, is way beyond any knowledge that can be expressed outwardly. You just know."

Indeed. I know.

The baby moved, and had times of expansion and times of a more hibernated state, where she'd tuck inward. However, because of the operation, the baby had very little room to grow, and move, and as a result the pain the mother experienced routinely, could be sheer agony.

By this point, I had witnessed, and therefore learned that missed miscarriage, especially in CP/EG could happen even in late pregnancy, and I felt that at some point this mother's body would reclaim the child. For years at this point, she had failed to get any medical care or recognition of her pregnancy. The only thing she had been able to get was prescribed medication for pain management.

I palpated and listened for fetal tones over the course of many hours. In that time we talked and I did energy healing work, and womb massage. What I felt was definitely a moving, living, very tiny baby. The child responded to my touch, and my presence. I could hear in the doppler her movement as she swirled around in the amniotic fluid. I could not pick up on consistent fetal tones, but the consistent movement and presence of a baby was definitely there.

One absolutely powerful, and central thing that I have learned over the course of my journey with CP/EG is this: Women's bodies and our babies, are wise, beyond wise beyond wise. Our ability to cope under impossible circumstances is phenomenal, even other-worldly. I remember praying and meditating inwardly during the whole appointment and visit. I came to the conclusion that this woman's body and baby know what they're doing. They had experienced trauma, rejection and neglect, and aside from the complications of pain and discomfort for her, she was in good health otherwise. The baby had obviously been experiencing terrible restrictions in her ability to grow and progress, but I felt intuitively, very profoundly, that she was on her own timetable. If no physical complications have arisen for the mother regarding the pregnancy, except the pain, for this long, we'd better take our cues from her body and baby, and not the other way around.

Sometimes there's nothing to do in these circumstances but to take it day by day, and stay dedicated to intuition. The Western scientific methodology is presently totally devoid of trust in the unknown, and therefore, the central, mystical aspects of Life Itself, and the Feminine Mysteries.

The Sacred Feminine, and Traditional Midwife's Art of Knowing, Without Outward Recognition

One of my greatest triumphs as a traditional midwife continues to go unclaimed and unrecognized with the mother. However, in the last few years I have come to deeply understand, and therefore embody the Sacred Feminine Art of Knowing, and "holding space," even while outwardly, there is denial and unrecognition.

The mother, when she conceived was very young, and the

circumstances surrounding the conception of her baby were extremely tumultuous and traumatic. I remember even before she was willing to accept her pregnancy due to negative tests, I remained confident in my own intuitive confirmation, and examination of her pregnancy symptoms.

I remember feeling her pregnant uterus, and being able to pick up on her baby's heartbeat through a fetoscope at around four months pregnant.

Her entire CP/EG experience would last fifteen months. I was there to track her pregnancy for the vast majority of that time, and I can testify to the fact that there was slow, but steady growth and movement the entire time.

What is the most painful part of all, is having been there for the entire pregnancy, and bonding with her baby, when nobody believed her and she had no one to turn to, only to have her not only doubt, but throw out her entire experience, and me with it. The main reason being, she desperately wanted to "normalize" her life with her boyfriend and presumed father of the child, and so any knowledge or discussion about the deeply mystical, and unknown aspects of her CP/EG, would definitely not be welcomed in that respect.

Around the ninth month of her CP/EG, she wanted me to listen with a doppler, and I had intuitively bought one for the first time, specifically for her pregnancy.

Before I go to examine any mother and baby, I am given permission of course from the mother herself, but I also ask permission from the baby. This time with the doppler, I asked permission, and I prayed, asking the baby to show himself for the sake of his mother, for she desperately needed that more outward, obvious confirmation. It took I think about twenty-minutes, resting every few minutes from the prodding with the doppler. Finally, way, way down deep inside the mother's pelvis, we found a consistent, strong and oh! So beautiful, baby heartbeat! It was a celebration, an absolutely joyous occasion!

She would go on to get full medical confirmation, and I would walk with her still through the remaining months of her pregnancy, providing prenatal care. She would give birth to her healthy, beautiful son at a hospital, and I would attend, in the presence of medical professionals, as her doula. She gave birth completely naturally, and I was able to help guide her through the wild and intense dance of childbirth.

~~~

One of the first times I traveled as a doula to attend to a CP/EG mother was around six years ago. I paid almost completely out of pocket for that trip, but I remember feeling very called by the Spirit to make the trip. My husband, and my second CP/EG baby, who was around one-year-old, traveled with me.

It was so early on in the work, I really didn't know what to expect, but I continued to pray and meditate with every step, and even, or especially when things just seemed totally bewildering and mysterious, I consistently received that I am the woman CP/EG women need. I just knew I needed to totally trust in that knowing-the suffering of women in this realm was, and continues to be so great.

It was one of the first times I'd palpated the uterus of a CP/EG mother, who'd been experiencing her pregnancy for at least six months, with very little growth, and rather bewilderingly, ambiguous symptoms.

I'd had two CP/EG babies at that point, but both had grown consistently in the womb, even if it was slower at times than most babies. I knew at least that these babies could be very tucked in, and very private about their presence in the world.

I decided to pray for a gentle, but grounding hand when it came to this mother's rather anxious energy surrounding her experience, not to mention the upheaval it was causing in her marriage.
~~~

I first tried to listen with a fetoscope but couldn't hear anything. So I began to gently palpate, asking for permission to enter her baby's space. After a few minutes, the baby came to my hand. I remember it was a very small baby, but they definitely responded to my touch, and I remember the mother crying because it was the first time she'd been able to really feel consistently the baby's movements, while I gently stimulated her uterus, and pressed on the baby. Later, I also listened with my doppler, and I remember the mother and I correlating together what she was feeling from the baby, and the movements of the baby I was simultaneously picking up from the doppler. I was inspired to ask her if she'd been able to feel her little boy who was at the time around two years old, in utero. She said that it had been difficult. She could only feel him if she breathed a certain way, and sat in a certain position.

The vast majority of CP/EG mothers and babies who reached out to me for support and advice in the first four to five years, would not be able to carry their babies to term. The reasons I began to understand deeply were profoundly connected to shame, neglect, and abuse.

Recently I discovered an article published by a mainstream pop-medical website who brazenly makes the albeit, casually-toned claim, stating as if the "overall medical community at large" has been able to make the connection between Cryptic Pregnancy and neonaticide. I know for a fact that there has been no such connection made medically, however, in my work I have written and/or spoken of extensively the risk of mothers killing their babies in utero through substance abuse and neglect-and cryptic pregnancy.

~~~~

The "hijacking" of vital forces, mentally, emotionally, and physically that I have witnessed in my life in Modern Women and culture, has been an overwhelming, impressive, and devastating thing to behold.
~~~~

One of the terrible symptoms of this "hijacking" is the conscious, and/or unconscious, definitely compulsive need to deny, seemingly at all costs, what is *real*; and instead embrace, and even pour vitality into what is not only false, but even aggressively destructive- especially to the women themselves.

Routinely for example, Modern Women, at the risk (and cost) of their lives, enter into relationships with men, who are unknown to them in character, and yet; they plunge headlong into routine sexual relations - often consumed by alcohol intake or other substances. All the while telling themselves, and others, that this is "liberated, free behavior." When in fact, it's terribly dangerous emotionally, and oftentimes physically.

I have seen this pattern similarly in the way CP/EG women (and other women), will be so desperate to maintain their sense of control in their particular social and familial circles; they prefer to over-pay, entrust, and even obey the directives, minimalistic attitudes, and flaky services of "experts," such as many medical professionals or Instagram-Success "Alternative" Birthworkers; to the detriment, and even fatality of themselves and/or their babies in utero; than acknowledge that I have been the only one able to help them, in a substantial way. Most, end up veering off the rails of their own lives- oftentimes going against, or refusing to acknowledge my proven, sound advice, experience, and insight.

PART FOUR

My Traditional and Medical Treatments and Suggestions

This section is general guidance for healing and correcting the root causes of fertility/reproductive issues in women, including CP/EG women; and I have added/curated sections specifically for guiding women in CP/EG.

You've been having difficulty getting pregnant. Or maybe there were issues during pregnancy that were not addressed properly, and perhaps, led to miscarriage. What do you do now? We've been there; the doubting, the confusion, and even the deep fear. One thing that I can tell you is that as a mother, an intuitive healer, a doula, and a midwife, having worked with hundreds of women experiencing fertility issues of all kinds from all over the world over the last fifteen years- as well as having my own fertility struggles- it's that, fertility is not in itself a complicated issue, but emotionally, psychologically, and spiritually, it can be very complex; and lead to difficulty, and need for healing within the body.

For you, the first thing to do Mama, is to find calmness and return to your center. We will discuss the physical action steps to take soon, such as herbal and nutritional care; but to begin, I cannot stress enough the importance of reducing anxiety and getting out of the fight-or-flight state.

In my experience, the primary reason for all of the stress and confusion that typically surrounds fertility in modern culture, is the lack of integration within the psyche, in relation to the body. With our overall culture, and medical influences, more often than not, pulling our attentions away from the answers within, and insisting that the answers to our problems lie in outside endorsements; well, it is no wonder even experts are admitting that our stress levels overall as a society, are causing enormous problems regarding our health, especially our fertility.

This means that all of the different aspects of the mind, emotions and physical body, as well as the opinions of society, the healthcare system, and even family or friends, are in a heightened state of conflict, contradiction, severe doubt or disbelief, and even disassociation or denial. The mother who is experiencing this can easily be overwhelmed by this chaotic energy that is within her and around her...and of course especially, her growing child in the womb.

While we may or may not be able to change the surrounding environment, we can always make changes within our self. You can take the reigns of your life and be the one that decides how you will progress and grow; and a lot of that is going to depend firstly, on your ability to relinquish control to your body's innate wisdom.

The steps I am going to take you through here are going to touch on every level of being; the spiritual/soulful, emotional, psychological and physical.

The First Step

Finding Your Center, Becoming Calm and Grounding

Centering With Your Breath

Learning to focus on your breathing and quieting your mind is often the first step to integrating, and being open to new, and unexpected possibilities in your life. It will begin the process of helping your energy, hormones, emotions, and thoughts to become more peaceful and harmonized.

Here is a simple but powerful exercise that I have suggested many times to mothers:

Start by sitting crossed legged on the floor in a quiet space and begin to focus on your breath.

Put your hands on your abdomen and feel the gentle movement of your belly as you breathe.

Visualize energy flowing through your pelvis and going straight down into the earth. This flow of energy is called "Grounding" and can help calm the lower Chakras (Energy Centers) to bring you out of survival mode and fear responses.

Feel the calming rhythm of your breath. It's the same rhythm that your baby is (or will be) listening to. Begin to search for the feeling of your baby, (spiritually or physically), sensing their presence and their budding energy.

Now, take a deep breath in through your nose. When you exhale, focus on surrendering and accepting what is happening in your life right now. Pay attention to the parts of you that are still fighting. There may be some aspects of your psyche that are in a state of disbelief, confusion, fear, helplessness and/or anger around why this is happening to you. Perhaps the rational part of your mind craves evidence, as well as tangible, and immediate answers about what you are experiencing. Remind yourself that not all things in life have clear answers and simply take time to find and resolve.

Continue to practice acknowledging the emotions that arise, whatever they are. Let yourself be in the present moment with these thoughts and feelings, and give yourself permission to feel doubt or excitement. Oftentimes, by giving yourself a chance to explore and begin to understand what you are feeling, and where it is coming from is enough to begin to calm the turbulent waters of emotion.

Continue this meditative technique for ten minutes. Set a timer and allow yourself to Be, if only for that long. Repeat this on a daily basis, whenever you get a moment, or when you go to lie down at night.

We are sometimes thrown into a situation that forces us to wake up and evolve. For many women, this may be the first time in their lives that they are brought through such an intimate journey with the deepest parts of themselves. At the heart of becoming an integrated person who finds balance within this process, is the ability to Trust Your Intuition. *My dearest one, there is no way around this but through the inner voice.*

Remember that Life Itself is Good, and its ancient principles work, and much, much deeper than that, Life Itself can be trusted. It may at times seem against you, and maybe there are times ourselves, other people, or circumstances are against us- but to remember that at the center of Life's Core Principles; where there is Life there is Death/Endings, and where there is Death there is Life/Rebirth- is to tap into a timeless reality within; that no matter what is happening on the outside, this timeless reality never loses hope, and is constantly open to new, and ever-evolving possibilities and experiences.

The Second Step

Physical Needs and Nourishment for Fertility

Basic Principles

There are primarily three principles that need to be consistently addressed in fertility, that ultimately address women's overall health, and they are the following:

1. Increasing Circulation to the Pelvis
2. Toning and Strengthening the Uterus
3. Growth and Nourishment for You and Baby

A nutrient dense diet is absolutely necessary in this process and in life in general. In fact, with a nutrient-dense diet, the herbal treatments are far more effective.

If these areas are weakened or deficient, a baby may struggle to thrive; and in my experience, this is becoming more and more common. If these areas are addressed, the likelihood of having a healthy pregnancy increases significantly.

Ignoring significant health issues or continuing unhealthy lifestyle habits contributes to preventing the body from being able to efficiently support the growing child. Under these conditions, the body will struggle to maintain the pregnancy, hormonal balance, and the woman's overall health.

The Third Step

Pregnancy Herbal Support & Nutrition

Nature's Gifts and Our Ancestors' Wisdom

The herbs will be listed according to these three vital categories for pregnancy, and overall health:

Circulation

Toning and Strengthening
Growth and Nourishment

Many of the herbs/supplements will have multiple benefits beyond the category by which I organize them. I'll make suggestions for dosages and frequency of which to take them.

You can mix and match the herbals, creating your own personal toolbox for health. Just be sure to choose at least one herb from each category and take them consistently.

Always stay in touch with your intuitive sense and listen to how the body is responding to what to take into your body and how. If you have any questions please email me, I am happy to help. (Contact Anshin B. at: <u>intuitivehealthmovement@gmail.com</u>)

Circulation

"Healthy blood nourishes every cell in the body. It flows through the body like a river, transporting essential nutrients and collecting waste. It ensures every tissue, organ and system has the fuel it needs. However, the pervasive nature of blood means that, once it is imbalanced, the whole body is imbalanced. Blood not only transports nutrients around the body, it also transports toxins. So care must be taken to ensure your blood has the purity, balance, and vitality your body needs for optimal health."

Referenced From

http://joyfulbelly.com

Motherwort Tincture
Suggested dosage: Five drops under tongue, in water or juice once a day, three days a week.

Iron Rich Foods
The CP/EG mother's body, as spoken of earlier, is in a state of "seizure." The ability to produce and sustain what is needed hormonally, in the cardiovascular, general metabolic, nervous and reproductive systems, has been greatly reduced, and a "hyper-rationing" has begun. There is often a loss of blood (monthly/periodic bleedings), yet the mother's uterus is often unable to form and grow in a normal way around the baby; and so the body is struggling not only to produce new blood cells, but also retain blood as well. This is one of the primary reasons why HCG and progesterone- two main hormones that create a healthy, vital endometrium lining, placenta, and sustain the process of proper fetal development- are unable to accumulate properly in the mother's system.

The primary issue with mainstream iron supplements is the inability for the body to absorb them. Here are some suggestions that have high metabolization, and can help effectively build the body's ability to build, sustain, and cleanse the cardiovascular system- and therefore the functionality of the womb- the baby's home:

Yellow Dock Tincture
Suggested dosage: One dropper under the tongue, in water or juice twice a week

Alfalfa Tincture
Suggested Dosage: One dropper per dose twice a day

Beets
Eat at least four servings of beets a week.

Whole Grains
Eat at least four servings of whole grains per week.

Spinach
Eat at least four servings of fresh, raw and/or steamed spinach per week. Or other dark, leafy greens.

Fresh Cooked Meat
Eat at least three servings of fresh cooked: Beef, Fish, or Pork per week.

Turmeric
I don't recommend using the capsule form. Take it as a powder and/or a tincture.

Suggested dosage for powder form: One tablespoon four times a week.

Suggested dosage for tincture form: Four drops under tongue, in juice or water four times a week.

Shepherd's Purse Tincture
Suggested dosage: One dropper once a day.

This particular herb is particularly powerful in helping the body retain the blood it creates and circulates. This helps the body heal, strengthen and nourish the womb and baby, keep Mama healthy, as well as create and retain necessary hormones.

Tonifying and Strengthening

The entire reproductive area is essentially the baby's home. It will carry, protect, nurture, and ultimately bring your baby out that cozy home and into your arms. Herbs work from within by providing your body with nutrients, minerals, and organic compounds that can activate hormones and create balance. This type of strengthening is a preventative and the effects gradually accumulate overtime, just like building a muscle; and quite literally, building and toning the muscles of the uterus and around the entire reproductive area.

By strengthening the uterus, it will help it be more effective in all of its responsibilities. It can also help make labor easier and contractions more effective when that time comes. A strong uterus creates a powerful foundation for your birth, labor and pregnancy.

Infusions

Infusions are a wonderful method of preparing herbs, utilizing and enhancing their effectiveness. It tends to make the herbal properties easier to metabolize.

How to Make An Infusion

1. Boil a quart of purified water
2. Take one handful of loose leaf herb and put it in an empty quart jar.
3. Fill with boiling water, cap and let sit for 2+ hours.
4. Decant, add honey if desired and drink.

Raspberry Leaf Infusion
Suggested dosage: At least 1.5 cups daily

Nettle Leaf Infusion
Suggested dosage: At least one cup daily

Red Clover Infusion
Suggested dosage: At least 1.5 cups daily

Comfrey Leaf Infusion

Susun Weed is an internationally renowned herbalist who recommends comfrey leaf infusions for their safety and effectiveness. I have had a lot of positive experience with comfrey leaf as well. There is a lot of misleading information about comfrey out there, so I want to tell you that the leaf infusion is incredibly nourishing and beneficial during pregnancy and in general. And as with any herb, It must be treated with respect and approached with knowledge and intuition.

There is an abundance of minerals, folic acid and protein that are available when comfrey leaf is assimilated in its infusion form. It is most effective when taken consistently for promoting elasticity and tone within the uterus and pelvis. It can also provide excellent nourishment for the bones.

Suggested dosage: At least one cup daily

Calcium

Calcium is considered a "health tonic" in the Wise Woman Tradition of healing and midwifery because of its vital role in literally creating a stable and healthy core for much of the tissue and blood cells of the body, particularly in the reproductive organs.

The best way to take calcium is through calcium-containing foods. This is because calcium is not absorbed by the body without the presence of certain vitamins and minerals. Foods that are rich in calcium tend to contain all of those necessary vitamins and minerals. On average a woman needs to consume around 1000-2000 mg of calcium daily. *This is especially important in pregnancy.*

Great Sources of Calcium include any variety of seaweed, particularly kelp, dark leafy greens and fish.

One of my very favorite healers of The Wise Woman Tradition Susun S. Weed states in her book, "Wise Woman Herbal for the Childbearing Year:"

"There are roughly 200 grams of calcium in two ounces of nuts (excluding peanuts), one ounce of dried seaweed, two ounces of carob powder, one ounce of cheese, half a cup of cooked greens (kale, collards, dandelion especially), half a cup of milk, three eggs, four ounces of fish, or one tablespoon of molasses."

"Shepherd's purse is beneficial for everyone though, not just women in childbirth or those prone to nosebleeds. This mild member of the mustard group is high in oxytocin, contains more calcium per 100g than milk, and has all the factors needed for calcium absorption. The entire plant is edible. The fresh leaves and flowers are wonderful in salads, and can also be dried and added to soups and stews. The heart-shaped seed pods are delicious, and look adorable sprinkled on top of flat bread or pizza, or even as a topping for cupcakes and other desserts."
- Women'sHeritage.com

Dandelion Greens Tincture
Suggested dosage: Three droppers per day twice a week

Kelp Tincture
Suggested dosage: Three droppers per day twice a week

Fruit Sources
Dried dates, figs, prunes, papaya, raisins and elderberries.

Supplemental Sources

I recommend powder shakes, with a hearty blend of greens.

Nourishment and Growth

Everything we've been talking about so far is absolutely instrumental to you and your baby's nourishment and growth. I'm now going to focus on a specific aspect of nourishment, something that we call "stoking the inner fire" of the body and is the foundation of healthy hormonal function.

Without this attention to the "inner fire" of the cells, your blood has little to carry to the womb, the baby, the heart, brain and whole body. This type of nourishment ties everything together:

Good Fats and Oils

Dates
Suggested serving: Two large dates a day, three days a week

Avocados
Suggested serving: Two avocados a week

Flax Seed
Suggested serving: Three tablespoons of ground flaxseed a day, twice a week.

Coconut Oil
Suggested serving: Two tablespoons a day, three days a week

Hemp Seeds
Suggested serving: One tablespoon a day, four days a week

Nuts

All nuts contain good fats and oils. Eating a few every couple hours helps to effectively regulate the endocrine system, calm stress responses and sooth the nervous system.

Other suggested serving: Half a cup of nuts per day, three days a week.

Fish

I am part Japanese and we have some the oldest living people on earth. I think that there are many things that contribute to this awesome phenomenon, but the health and vitality of my people is related to the amount of fish we eat. We eat it cooked in so many different ways; Soup, marinated, grilled, baked and yes, raw!

Raw eaten fish is also known as "sashimi." (obviously very high-grade and very fresh, DO NOT eat raw fish, sashimi, at a dive-bar sushi place or at the mall. Only eat home-made with fresh, sashimi-grade fish, and/or quality restaurants where you're going to have to commit a few more dollars than usual to purchase sashimi). In Western medicine I was warned profusely about the *dangers* of eating my traditional, cultural food. Just like there is are all kinds of "medical" write-ups online about the "dangers" of herbs.

Please hear me out when I say; Over-simplifying *anything* and having a fear-based philosophy about our health and our bodies is bound only to get us in trouble and make us dependant on people we deem "higher" or more "educated" and/or more knowledgeable than us about our own bodies. Learning from others is essential but, total dependency and no self-education can lead to deepening ignorance and a destructive form of dependrency.

That being said, I believe that really good and superbly fresh raw fish, has potent and deeply nourishing good fats and oils that can support a pregnancy. I *craved* sashimi with at least a couple of my pregnancies and my children have always been incredibly healthy and strong. My "inner fires" in the womb, digestion, heart and brain kept burning with this aspect of my diet. My little "bun in the oven," in particular, my cryptic pregnancy and extended gestations flourished and thrived in that natural and necessary heat.

Suggested serving: Eat fresh fish (cooked, or not, to your liking) for at least three meals a week

One of my favorite ways to "stoke the feminine fires of creation:"

A quick word on caffeine. Caffeine is not generally seen in traditional medicine to be innately bad and/or dangerous to our bodies or babies. Like most things, it has its purpose in our health and enjoyment. In many cultures in Asia and Africa, "Chai" which base is black tea, is infused with herbs and some kind of fat, usually cream/butter and/or ghee (clarified butter) and consumed to "light a fire in the belly, heart and mind."

In women, in our wombs and ovaries, the central fires of creation. *In the West, caffeine drinks are consumed in excess with a crazy amount of processed sugar and artificial sweeteners. It's easy to see how different this form of caffeine consumption is from traditional caffeinated brews. This kind of dietary habit is detrimental to your health.*

The key is the use of wisdom and intuition that is cultivated through education; of the self, and from experienced healers.

Having said all that, the bases of the drinks that I will describe now are **coffee** and

black tea:

Serving suggestions:

Black tea: 12 ounces of boiling water per one tea bag
Coffee: 12 ounces of boiling water per four tablespoons of ground coffee

So this is how I do it:

Use a twelve ounce mason jar (a pint). Put one tea bag/tablespoon of loose-leaf or four tablespoons of ground coffee. Infuse either one with a couple (mix and match, get in touch with your inner herbalist/Wise Woman/alchemist) of the following by adding: ***Note, ginger and nettles help to nourish the adrenal glands which are central to the production as well as storage of energy and bring balance to the healthy, but nonetheless stimulative quality of the caffeine.***

1. A couple of black peppercorns
2. A teaspoon of fresh or ground turmeric
3. A teaspoon of ground, food-grade green powder and/or loose-leaf (spirulina, algae, spinach, parsley etc.). If you're using an extract either in powder form or liquid form, use less.
4. Pinch of cayenne pepper
5. A teaspoon of fresh or ground ginger
6. Cinnamon; One stick or one teaspoon+ of powder
7. Dandelion root
8. Honey
9. Cardamom
10. Dried mushroom, powder or pieces (I recommend Chaga Mushroom)
11. Nettles, tablespoon+ of loose leaf and only a few drops of the tincture. If you feel to add a little more of either, go ahead. It is very nourishing overall.

Fill to the top with boiling water, cap and let steep for around 15 to 25 min. (steep less if you wish to control the caffeine intake. You can also use less of the coffee or tea.

Strain and add a little raw sugar, agave syrup or honey if you haven't already. And for the **crowning and very important touch; add a teaspoon+ of any of the following:**

1. Unsalted butter

2. Coconut oil
3. Ghee
4. Cream
5. Whole milk
6. Hemp milk
7. Cashew milk

***I wouldn't recommend almond milk here because it tends to be less concentrated with good fats and oils with more of an emphasis on the protein content and the fats and oils are essential to "bringing the inner heat."**

Drink slowly, preferably seated, and enjoy!

Herbs and Medicinals for Healing Hormones

These herbs and medicinals are *more potent* and direct in nature than most of the herbs and foods listed in this write-up, which is why they have their own category. This section will focus on the direct treatment of the endocrine system which is responsible for the complex, beautiful and absolutely necessary function of the hormones.

Hormones are the physical link to our *feeling and emotional life*; sexually, emotionally, psychologically and spiritually. They connect us to the feelings in of all the systems in the body. Without proper function, everything begins to lose connection and we become ungrounded or uprooted from our physical bodies.

Vitex Tincture (Chaste Tree)
Suggested dosage: Four drops once a day up to seven days a week.

Liferoot Tincture
"Small doses of this tincture (3-8 drops a day), taken at least 14 days out of the month, will regulate hormone production, increase libido, normalize the menses, relieve menstrual pain, and improve fertility. The closely related Senecia jacobea and Senecio vulgaris can also be used." Susun Weed http:// www.susunweed.com/Article_Fertility_Herbs.htm

Partridge Berry Tincture
(Mitchella Repense)
Suggested dosage: Five drops a day up to seven days a week

Vitamin E
Vitamin E is said by traditional midwives to stabilize the fetus' attachment in the womb. I have found it is very beneficial all throughout CP/EG (the earlier it is taken the better), and the reason being; through the stabilization of the placenta and the revitalizing of the endometrium lining which Vitamin E provides, also helps, in the long run, boost more efficient hormone production overall. This includes especially HCG.

Suggested dosage: 500 IU per dose, up to twice a week

An Introductory Guide to Nutrition

Regimen, Suggestions and Needs:

Taking SoTru Nutrition Powder

Taking 1 scoop of the powder per day, along with the nourishing/healing foods below is going to be a great supplement to help more quickly stabilize your system, and make sure you get the complete nutrition needed daily. You can find it here:

SoTru Powder is available at most health food stores and Amazon.

Herbal Teas: Many are rich in so many vitamins, minerals and chlorophyll as well as other building blocks the body needs. To get the most out of them, take four tea bags (the same kind of tea) and put them into a quart jar and pour boiling water to the top of the jar. Cap, and let it steep for at least two hours.

Use the herbal infusion to add to soup, or just drink it as a tea, cold or hot, add it to smoothies, or sauces etc.

Some herbal teas to use: Nettle leaf, oatstraw, raspberry leaf, red clover, and corn silk. Tea brands to find these in: Traditional Medicinals and Celebration Herbals and Yogi Teas. If you can find other brands that's great! Go for it!

These are the nutrients we want to make sure we

incorporate into your food daily; here are some of the benefits and necessities of each one:

Greens, chlorophyll:
Purifies the blood and balances body ph. (this will also support the healthy production of blood, and therefore hormones.

Probiotics:
Live good bacteria that is responsible for building good digestion, metabolizing food, and keeping the immune system strong.

Enzymes:
Also responsible for digestion, metabolizing and immunity.

Good fats and oils:
Vital to cell health all throughout the body. Particularly nutrient to glands and gut lining.

Prebiotics:
Are fiber. They support gut health (the gut is central to immunity and emotional well being in addition to food digestion and assimilation). Fiber massages the gut, and keeps it vital by stimulating live bacteria.

Water! Water! Water!:
Adult Human Beings are around 60% water. Humans are also highly electromagnetic. Our physical and emotional energy and well-being rely on how much we are able to collect and conduct electromagnetic energy; from the Earth! Our electromagnetic fields are conducted and sustained through the water we replenish in our bodies. *Add sea salt and lemon to water for better absorption, just sea salt is also ok. Drink half your body weight in Oz. For example, I weigh 155 lbs, divide that by two, 77, therefore, around 77 oz. of water I need to drink per day.

Minerals:
Maintain bones, blood pressure/health, hormonal and emotional health (again, some of the many, many functions). _Minerals are central to the making of hormones!_

Vitamins:
Are essential to building and maintaining bones, muscles, making blood cells as well as many, many other functions.

Ideas for SoTru powder shake/smoothie ingredients:

Bananas: Rich in good fats, and vitamins.

Whole Milk Yogurt: Rich in calcium, probiotics and good fats.

Berries: Rich in antioxidants and other properties such as vitamins that keep cells healthy and heal damaged cells; blueberries, strawberries, goji berries etc. _I have personally experienced many times the effectiveness of consuming berries and reducing all manner of disordered symptoms within the uterus, such as: Inflammation and overall anemia._

Nut Butters: Cashew, almond, (if you're going to use peanut butter try to use a more natural brand; the mainstream brands tend to lack quality, but can still be a good source of protein). Nut butters have good fats and protein.

Breakfast Foods

Eggs (with yolk): Good fats, protein, try to get "cage free" or organic.

Butter: Good fats-_IMPORTANT:_ Avoid margarine and butter alternatives!

Whole grain cereals (not Kelloggs, too much sugar, artificial colors and preservatives). Some brands that use more raw, less processed ingredients are: Barbara's, Bob's Red Mill, Cascadian Farms, EnviroKidz. (Fiber, vitamins, minerals).

Bread: Buy whole grain bread or sprouted grain bread, sprouted grain bread brand: Ezekiel

Lunch and Dinner:

Whole grain brown rice (fiber, vitamins and **iron**).

Meats with no artificial growth hormones (good fats, protein, **iron**).

Bacon Get "uncured" bacon, which has no chemicals. (good fats, protein).

Sea Salt Minerals!

Greens Make sure the leafy greens are darker green, the darker the color, the more nutrients (**also good iron content**).

Add lots of orange vegetables and different colored vegetables to your cooking. Steam and/or fry lightly in olive oil or coconut oil, to maintain color because of nutrients. If you're going to boil, make sure you use the water from the boiled veggies because all the nutrients go in there when boiled.

Onions, garlic, apple cider vinegar, coconut oil, sesame oil, green herbs, spices: Maintains and builds immunity, keeps cells healthy, keeps digestive juices happy/flowing.

Bone Marrow broth Excellent for building good blood and all other cells: Boil whole chicken or pork with bones or beef with bones until very soft and the broth is very oily and rich. Use the broth to make soup, boil pasta (pasta will soak up the broth), cooked veggies etc.

Pasta Whole grain pasta: Fiber, vitamins, **iron.**

Fermented food Pickles with no added nitrates; Pickled cucumbers, cabbage, beets. Miso paste is fermented soybeans and excellent for immune and digestive health, "raw" cheese is made of raw milk which is full of good fats, enzymes and probiotics.

Popcorn Get non GMO if possible, with sea salt only (excellent fiber), or make it yourself on the stovetop: Add olive oil and/or nutritional yeast.

Here are some ingredients that are rich in vitamins and/or minerals, and/or complete proteins, and/or greens that I add to my sauces, pancake batter, and oil and vinegar dressings, soups and/or pasta and dishes in general:

- Nutritional Yeast
- Extra Virgin Olive Oil
- Coconut oil
- Liquid Aminos
- Dolce (seaweed flakes)
- Other plain, dried seaweed.
- SoTru Green Powder
- Herbs! (Sage, Parsley, Rosemary, Thyme, Dill etc)

Raw honey Full of nutrients that support the whole system; this is excellent for liver function, and therefore vital to blood health, circulation, and hormone production.

My Medical Suggestions

1. Since accumulation, production and retention of proper, healthy fluids in a CP/EG mother seems to be difficult, I suggest, if one is able, to receive IV hydration fluids every few months. It is vitally important to do this ONLY in *addition* to a conscious healthy diet, and assimilating many of my natural/alternative/traditional suggestions above. Under the right circumstances, and relationship with one's physician, this treatment can be obtained without medical confirmation of a pregnancy.

2. An ultrasound exam will most likely be considered "negative" if #1: A woman's pregnancy blood test comes back "negative," and/or #2: There is not a normal-sufficient amount of amniotic fluid around the growing baby to allow for the proper outward growth of the belly and baby. I highly suggest:

- *Very Important: Having Patience!* We are often in this situation because our bodies are refusing to be "pushed around," anymore; by our past and/or current harmful life experiences and decisions- no matter how unavoidable or unconscious they may have been.

- There is no time like the present, to make a close re-examination of our inward, outward, dietary, and all-around relational lives: Begin by educating yourself about herbal, traditional and alternative healing, and set yourself on a plan/regimen.

- When women actually set themselves on a self-informed, intuitive health-plan, I have enough experience to know that *doors open:* Their body proceeds with the pregnancy in a healthy manner, or their body passes on the pregnancy through miscarriage, and returns to normal; or, sometimes, the women are able receive medical confirmation down the line.
- The correlation between the production and accumulation of amniotic fluid, and the accumulation and production of HCG and other hormones is, in my experience, central, and vital to tracking the health of a CP/EG;
- In some circumstances, especially when a woman follows my herbal and dietary suggestions, she is able to obtain a positive lab and/ or ultrasound test.

3. **Lastly, as they say, *"be careful what you wish for, because you just might get it,"*** while medical confirmation of your pregnancy is overall, a good thing; it can also serve to totally undermine a woman's intuition and self-growth. As my chart clearly illustrates; the vast majority of instances where the healthy growth and birth of a CP/EG baby is prevented, has largely to do with the misplaced, over-medicalization of women and childbearing.

A Chart Illustrating My Associative Observations, and Experiential Data on CP/EG

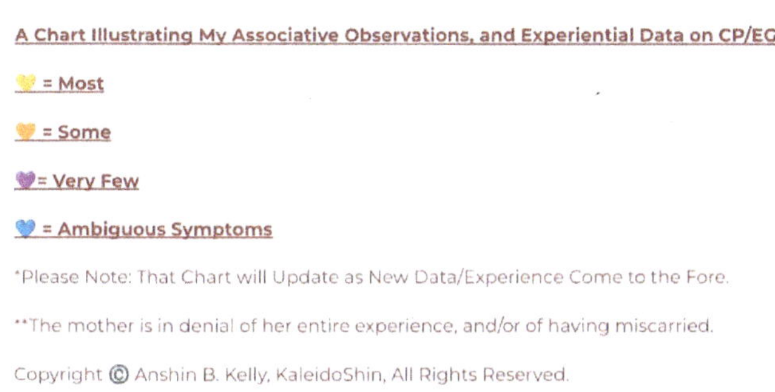

CP/EG Mothers Overall Health History and Experience	CP/EG Mother Gave Birth: Naturally/Medically	CP/EG Mother: Miscarried	CP/EG Mother: Miscarried and Remained in Denial**
Reproductive Trauma	🧡	💛	🧡
Cesarean Section(s)	🧡	💛	🧡
Getting Pregnant Soon after Birth	🧡	💛	🧡
Bleeding while Pregnant	🧡	💛	🧡
CP/EG After Tubal Ligation	🧡	💛	💛
CP/EG After Artificial Insemination	🧡	💛	💛
Emotional/Sexual/Mental Trauma	💜	💛	🧡
Other Trauma/Surgeries	💜	💛	🧡
Cancer Treatment/Other	💜	💛	🧡

Medical Treatments for Physical Disease			
Getting Pregnant Using Condoms or other Protection	💜	💛	💛
Hormonal Birth Control	💜	💛	🧡
Medications	💜	💛	🧡
Emotional/Mental Instability	💜	💛	💛
Mental Illness (Observed or Medically Diagnosed)	💜	💛	💛
Sexually Indiscriminate	💜	💛	🧡
Abortions/Plan B	💜	💛	🧡
Unmarried	💜	💛	🧡
Father Absent/Abusive/Unsupportive	💜	🧡💙	🧡
Father Present and Supportive	🧡	💛	💜
Father Present and Unsupportive	💜	💛	💛
Alcohol/Substance Abuse	💜	💛	💛
Suicidal/Suicide	💜	💜	💜
Processed Diets/Lack of Nutrition	🧡	💛	🧡
Neglect/Ostracism/Humiliation	🧡	🧡	🧡
CP/EG Woman: Passive Aggressive, Verbally/Financially Abusive and Manipulative	💜	🧡💙	🧡

Has Faith/Spirituality	💛	🧡	💜
Resentful of Men	💜	🧡💙	🧡

The End

115

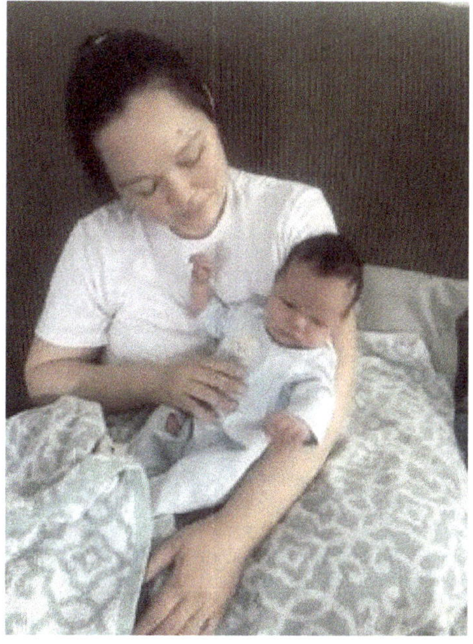

www.ingramcontent.com/pod-product-compliance
Lightning Source LLC
Chambersburg PA
CBHW070813260726

48660CB00005B/1841